Dreams ___Die Hard, *Truth*___ Sets Free

A TRIUMPH OF THE HUMAN SPIRIT

DAVE STONE

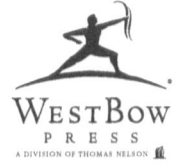

WESTBOW
PRESS
A DIVISION OF THOMAS NELSON

Scriptures taken from the Holy Bible, New International Version®, NIV®.
Copyright © 1973, 1978, 1984, 2011 by Biblica, Inc.™ Used by permission
of Zondervan. All rights reserved worldwide. www.zondervan.com The
"NIV" and "New International Version" are trademarks registered in the
United States Patent and Trademark Office by Biblica, Inc.™

Cover photos © Terri Stone

WestBow Press books may be ordered through booksellers or by contacting:

WestBow Press
A Division of Thomas Nelson
1663 Liberty Drive
Bloomington, IN 47403
www.westbowpress.com
1-(866) 928-1240

Because of the dynamic nature of the Internet, any web addresses or links contained in
this book may have changed since publication and may no longer be valid. The views
expressed in this work are solely those of the author and do not necessarily reflect the
views of the publisher, and the publisher hereby disclaims any responsibility for them.

Any people depicted in stock imagery provided by Thinkstock are models,
and such images are being used for illustrative purposes only.
Certain stock imagery © Thinkstock.

ISBN: 978-1-4908-0427-9 (sc)
ISBN: 978-1-4908-0428-6 (hc)
ISBN: 978-1-4908-0426-2 (e)

Library of Congress Control Number: 2013914441

Printed in the United States of America.

WestBow Press rev. date: 09/10/2013

TABLE OF CONTENTS

DEDICATION

This book is dedicated to:

Jesus Christ, for the many ways He has brought Terri through tribulations and made her more than a conqueror.

Mary Graterr, her Mother, for having faith in and working hard with her in the midst of many serious physical problems, to give her the opportunity for a reasonably normal life.

Doctor James Collins, for helping her through difficult situations, encouraging and providing her opportunities to stretch personally and professionally.

Dr. Stephen J. Suomi, who, by trusting, encouraging, assigning growing duties and allowing freedom to choose how to perform them, provided her incentives and opportunities to grow professionally. Her resultant growth has been much more than could have been expected.

Her brothers, for putting up with a bossy older sister who's many physical problems seriously impacted their lives, but generally provided needed love and friendship.

Those teachers, especially Betty Reid-Matthews, who looked past her problems, invested themselves in her, providing the teaching, friendship and encouragement to help her achieve far more than had been expected with her disabilities.

PREFACE

This series of little life stories started with a collection of memories on scraps of paper by my wife, Terri at the age of 14. She intended to write a book and name it Dreams Die Hard. Over the years the scraps were lost but not the intent to encourage other people, especially those with hidden disabilities, by writing her memories and experiences into a book.

About twenty years after starting to collect these memories we met and were married on September 26, 1992. Since I was blessed to have a school teacher mother with a love for the English language, extended to me, we have chosen to have me draw out those old memories and search old photos and records to write it.

During the research and hearing the daily experiences of Terri's life, I started to see the obvious spiritual aspects of the developing narrative. Clearly this was her terribly difficult emotional and spiritual journey with one of its main themes the contrast of her father's attempts to drown his disappointments in alcohol compared to Terri's continuing struggles to understand and deal with reality. It was this contrast, informed by my own spiritual experiences that brought out the rest of the book title, Dreams Die Hard <u>Truth Sets Free.</u>

The writing has been a matter of writing a little now and more later in no particularly organized way. It has been a work of at least ten years with parts of it recast and rewritten many times on old computers that I have hunted and pecked on with little understanding of how they worked or why they keep jumping the text around in their own mysterious ways. For example, the chapter headings are moved even after I have just carefully hit the save button to try and maintain chapter head space. It drives me crazy but here I am typing the preface on how the book got this far and I'm tempted to say "Darned if I know."

ACKNOWLEDGEMENTS

Pastor Fred Miller of Cumberland Valley Church of the Brethren in Christ in Dillsburg, Pennsylvania for editing.

A dear friend who wishes to remain anonymous for greatly encouraging publishing.

WestBow Press' staff for their guidance, patience, and assistance in publishing this book.

INTRODUCTION

This story of my wife's overcoming her many serious disabilities provides a peek at a life experience far different from most. It includes a first ten years of uncontrolled epileptic seizures and a variety of other major health problems. It also has molestation, suicide, a father's alcoholism, problems of IQ testing and failures of the school system. These factors and the gypsy lifestyle of the military including two assignments in Germany, combined to create the crazy, comical, and sad events of this dysfunctional family. Looking at it, she can see God's hand, providing helpers, guiding, comforting, and enabling her to overcome difficulties, although she didn't recognize it then.

It is written from the perspective that while our dreams are important and may lead to great success, there can be another side to the picture. It is based on her life with epilepsy and as the first child in a deeply dysfunctional family. Epilepsy has taught her to treasure the opportunity to think clearly and to try hard to understand what is real. It also caused her to be considered a strange child by others, especially youngsters her age. Partly, because of the loneliness this produces, she has a deep appreciation for human relationships, which hopefully shows in this book.

Today, although she still has many serious health problems, they appear to be manageable. Her greatest struggles are in dealing with old statements of some teachers, doctors and neighbors that she was a lost cause, who would never amount to anything. Especially painful and hard to deal with, was her father's agreement with that opinion and his lack of support. Her problems with other children, her father, teachers and doctors, supported her belief that if she wanted or needed anything, she would have to fight for it. Gradually, she has recognized that her accomplishments are much more than could be reasonably expected. This is helping her let go of the old negative attitudes that have haunted her. Also she has learned that other ways often work better than fighting. Old habits of thought die hard too, even the negative ones.

The book starts with a brief look at how her parents may have become who they were. It is based on what they said, her experiences with them and their parents, and from some old family photos and records. After all this time, the evidence of what happened before her birth is rather limited. This, along with the unusual dynamics of military family life may cause her opinions to be unfair in presenting her father, especially his feelings and motivations. She sincerely hopes not, because she always loved him, deeply desired his approval and doesn't want to defame his memory. However, she believes wholeheartedly in following where reality leads. It is important to remember that most of the reality presented here is from her mother's and her perspectives. This may be from their tight bonding and the stories her Mom used to tell. Also her place in a military family placed her closer to her mother's experience than her father's. The testing of the accuracy of this perspective came in her day to day living.

Although a number of parts of it are painful, she has attempted to give a truthful picture of their family life, as she witnessed it, while trying to somewhat moderate the effect on people mentioned. In order to achieve the desired moderation in the attempt to write a biography some names, places and details have been changed without altering the essential truths of events mentioned.

MY PARENTS

Dad's father had the reputation for being a hard man and a stern disciplinarian. Dad didn't seem to feel accepted by him. I have come to believe that Dad's apparently low self esteem and continuous drive to look good was an attempt to be accepted. His low self esteem appears to be a result of his relationship with his parents. His mother seemed a rather harsh woman who didn't express love very well. She'd lived a hard life, earning most of the family income while raising three children. Her husband, a hard drinker, worked occasionally. I doubt that she was able to provide Dad with enough emotional support. Also, Dad was the middle son and didn't have the advantage of the oldest child's experience or the attention usually reserved for the youngest. It is not unusual for a middle child to have difficulty establishing a comfortable role in the family.

I have a number of old photographs of Dad from childhood to adulthood. From them I've noticed that he smiles in very few of them. His facial expressions, especially around the eyes, seem to say, "Am I acceptable?" These pictures, along with his behaviors, support the impression that he was not comfortable with himself. Perhaps this was the major reason for his constantly trying to look good, and partly the source of his problem with alcoholism. Some of the problem of using alcohol or other substances to escape from the pains of life are that they become insulation from life's joys and stunt emotional growth. The escape produces a lot of unnecessary pain. It is noteworthy that Mom used to say that she had five children: my three brothers, me, and Dad, who had never grown up.

A family member with whom Dad grew up remembers him as a rollicking playboy. But with his alcohol problem, he gradually became a man who had to have his whiskey every night. Later in his marriage it was not unusual for him to finish the evening by passing out. One of my photographs is of him in a stupor at the dinner table with his face in his dinner dish. His drunkenness may have partly resulted from his inability to cope with my epilepsy. He told me that my epilepsy was the reason for his inability to advance in military rank. He said he would have had more opportunity for promotion if he'd been stationed where the fighting was. But my brother, Johan, told me at Dad's funeral that Dad had used my epilepsy to avoid being shipped to battle areas. It is much easier to blame everyone and everything than to take responsibility for what we do.

On the other hand, it may be that our need of him because of the extraordinary circumstances of my epilepsy truly was his reason for avoiding the fighting. If so, it would have been nice if he'd had the grace not to blame his failure on my epilepsy and, by implication, on me. This is especially true because his negative attitude toward his senior officers and his drinking were self destructive. For example, Mom told me about an occasion when Dad was stationed overseas. He phoned home to Mom for money to pay the cost of damages he owed for breaking things in a bar fight. This was not easy since military pay was not that great. Mom went to a bank and borrowed the money. It demonstrates his dependence on his wife. It was a dependence that he hated, but he demonstrated it over and over. Having other people clean up after him was not particularly rare. For example, rather than redeem his own bad checks, which he had passed out at liquor stores, he sent Mom or, when I was older, me. If he had a bad check at one store he would purchase his booze at others until Mom or I could cover the bad one.

Mom's father was a Navy man who was highly organized and precise in his personal life. Grandpa married a loving, emotionally strong, but physically delicate little woman. He bossed her around and abused her both emotionally and physically. At times when he was drunk Grandma poured his liquor down the sink. Grandpa became so angry that he hit Grandma; although this was an allegation that we couldn't prove. The only proof we had were the bruises on her arms that we believed came from him.

Mom was an intelligent, inventive, strong, resilient woman. With her quick wit she was very good at expressing her ideas and could skin you verbally if she chose. She attended William and Mary College where, during her sophomore year, she was courted by two students who both went on to have military careers. She chose Dad, another sophomore, after a rather short courtship. The man that she gave up for Dad went on to a more successful military profession, rising to the rank of colonel. I suspect that Dad, the rollicking play boy remembered by his relatives, loosened up with the aid of his bottle. He and Mom were such terrific ballroom dancers that when they danced other dancers left the floor and watched. They left William and Mary College after their sophomore year, married, and Dad joined the Army.

Over the years, I began to wonder what drew Mom and Dad together. The story of my parents' courtship and marriage had the elements of a strong woman and weak man, drawn to one another to fulfill their emotional needs, hers for control and his for support. Dad's being a 'good time Charley' kind of guy, his self doubts eased by his bottle and his undeniable dancing ability may have played a role in drawing them together. They were like Fred Astaire and Ginger Rogers on the dance floor. But, as enticing as this might have been for Mom, I suspect the vulnerability of his self doubts may have been even more magnetic. She was a personable and powerful young woman with great compassion and self confidence. She may have believed that her love and care would fix his underlying lack of self confidence.

Mom wanted a large family, so they started trying to have a child. But she had trouble, having several miscarriages before I was born. Conception continued to be difficult for her, and she continued to miscarry until after the birth of my sister, her fifth child, in Germany much later. Finally, after we returned to Augusta, Georgia, Mom's gynecologist told her that her reproductive system was worn out. She accepted his verdict and had the hysterectomy he recommended.

Dad was able to escape many of the pressures caused by the severity of my epilepsy and other frequent illnesses because he was at work and out of the house, even sometimes an ocean away. Mom, as the bulwark of our family, had to deal with all the family problems. After I became old enough, and my seizures were mostly under control, Mom sometimes sought temporary relief in the bottle. But this was not a regular thing and did not present the severe problems that accompanied Dad's continuous drinking.

MY FIRST FOUR YEARS

I was born in Augusta, Georgia, had a father in the Army, three younger brothers, and much later, a sister, who died of sudden infant death syndrome within her first three weeks. I was diagnosed with epilepsy when I was eight months old. Consciousness came and went as much as forty to sixty times daily for the first ten years of my life due to both grand mal and petit mal seizures. The seizures gradually decreased after that. However, this was not a straight-line decline, and there were a number of relapses. Grand mal happened much less frequently than petit mal. Grand mal produced convulsions with complete loss of consciousness and muscle control. Petit mal, while much more frequent, wasn't as dramatic. It brought shorter consciousness loss and only partial, but varied, muscle control loss. Naturally, I don't remember lots of things because of the seizures and the brain-numbing effects of the heavy drugs I needed to try to control the seizures.

The Army life meant frequent relocation to new base assignments. Some of the relocations may have been caused by Dad's drinking and his discomfort with and disrespect for authority. His army units may have transferred him to get rid of the problems he caused. With all the travel and my many illnesses,

I attended fourteen different schools by high school graduation, which took fourteen years.

I think doctors and my mother were the only people who fully grasped the severity of my epilepsy. She was the only person who witnessed and understood nearly all the consequences of my various maladies. Her substantial understanding of their effects on me was only possible because of the great love and mercy she felt for me as she witnessed my pains and struggles. It was almost like we were one person. This especially tight bond is a typical feature of dysfunctional families. Members have exaggerated and inappropriate roles that produce a lack of proper understanding of appropriate roles and boundaries between the family members. This inappropriate sense of reality comes from the enormous pressures caused by the power of the particular problem[s] they face. Children's failure to understand that the special realities of their lives are not the norm helps to cause a continual confusion in human relationships that is difficult to overcome even in adulthood.

My epilepsy may be partly the result of an inherited tendency for this brain malfunction. Dad, with his need to look good, claimed there was no record of epilepsy in his family, and any predisposition must come from Mom's family, which had no record of epilepsy. His seizures, which became apparent years after seizures appeared in three of his children, make his blaming Mom for a possible tendency appear especially nasty. If there was an inherited tendency, it probably came through him, and there does seem to be a likelihood of an inherited tendency since three of his children had epilepsy.

The medical record shows that my seizures started with a fall on my head from a bed in my eighth month. This was while we were living at the Vogelweh U. S. Army Base in Heidelberg,

Germany during Dad's first assignment there. The record shows that my eyes rolled back in my head, but I didn't lose consciousness, and was not taken to a doctor. During my ninth month I had several episodes a day. My eyes would roll back and head drop momentarily without apparently losing consciousness or falling. Then a large gap appears in the medical record. The next entry, in my eighteenth month, mentions a much more severe seizure. This happened after being seen at the Landstuhl U S Army Hospital, near Kaiserslautern for the rolling back of my eyes. They found fever and a slight ear infection, and referred me to neurology for later testing. On the way home to the US Army Vogelweh Base, from the hospital my fever increased to one hundred four degrees. Then I had my first grand mal convulsion. It lasted several minutes. Since the Vogelweh dispensary was much closer than Landstuhl, I was immediately seen at Vogelweh. From there, I was sent back to Landstuhl for evaluation. During this period the records show that I had upper respiratory infections, tonsillitis, skin rashes and an eye squint. I was a very sickly child, and maladies, as serious as pneumonia, were frequent visitors.

Toward the end of my first time in Germany, Mom received word that her mother was very ill and weak, unlikely to live without strong moral support and close family care. She was not eating. Mom and I flew to San Leandro, California to take care of her. It was there, that I first remember the joy of helping to take care of my charming Grandma. I made her toast, and was proud of being able to make it golden brown without burning it. Gradually, Mom's loving care and my little help nursed Grandma back to health, and we flew back to Germany.

FORT DOUGLAS, UTAH

When I was nearly five years old, Dad was transferred to Fort Douglas, Utah, where we attended Catholic Church. One Sunday Dad chose to attend church with the family (a very rare occurrence). We dressed in our best clothes as usual for church and arrived early. We entered the back of the church, trooped down the aisle all the way to the second row of pews and sat down. Shortly, the music started, the priest entered and started to speak. I stood up on the pew and said, "My Daddy says that no one talks in church." Dad was trying to shrink down into the pew while a quiet rustle of giggles came from the parishioners. The priest explained to me that he was supposed to conduct the service and continued with his message.

I was enrolled in kindergarten at Catholic school in nearby Salt Lake City. Learning was extremely difficult with consciousness coming and going, and with illnesses causing me to be often absent from school. When conscious, my life was experienced in a fog, caused by many heavy doses of medicine. This was necessary to get the little seizure control possible, with the best drug routines my doctors had been able to discover. Meanwhile, they kept looking for better combinations, amounts and timings of medications.

In school, I was the strange, spastic, new kid with the squint and skin rashes. As you may imagine, I was not welcomed with open arms by my fellow students. Young children, learning who they are and developing friendships with familiar children, are not good at welcoming strangers. This is especially true for one as odd as I must have seemed to them. Also, with my disability I was spoiled by Mom's very supportive attention and I expected the same interest and close attention at school. It was not to be; neither teachers nor other students were about to invest that much of themselves in this strange new creature. Teachers were too busy with other students to be able to do it. Children didn't have any desire to yield to my hunger for immediate attention. This reinforced my attitude of 'me against the world, which Mom may have started by telling me, "It's you and me against the world." I was a fighter, trying to defend what I considered my rights. As the years went by the roughest edges of this attitude were somewhat smoothed. But the struggles to have my natural talents recognized by teachers, the rest of the world and Dad reinforced my fighting inclinations. My many physical problems and aggressive attitude did not make talents easy to see.

One of the clearest examples of my lack of positive relationships with other students was the time I had a seizure, near the top of the school's second floor steps. I fell down the steps all the way to the first floor and had cuts and bruises. My books and papers were scattered all over. Another student was there, and when I asked him for help he said, "No." I was so angry because I thought he should have helped me that I socked him on the nose. His nose bled and he developed a black eye. This didn't help my relationships with students or teachers.

Many of my teachers were overwhelmed by the problems my presence created. Beside my aggressiveness, seizures and drug reactions, there were my fellow students' reactions to them. The combination was poorly suited to teaching. These events wore on teachers' patience, which sometimes showed in their attitudes toward me. The disorderly classroom situation made some teachers suggest my placement in a special class, or institutionalization. Unfortunately, special classes were not usually available; and thank God that Mom would not consider the institutional option. She believed in me, much more than I did, and I would not have developed as well without her constant love and encouragement. My life is owed to her. I believe the impatience of some of my teachers, has made me deeply appreciate patience, so that I have become more patient when teaching than I am in other situations.

Teachers had a lot to contend with then, as now, but more is known about epilepsy than years ago. Also, teachers have learned to accommodate disabled students more than ever since the American Disabilities Act. This federal law requires reasonable accommodation for the disabled. Seizures caused complete interruptions of thought, so I had to try to remember where I was in the thought process. I often forgot whether I was at home, school or somewhere else in my drugged fog. My consciousness was interrupted so often that I had to concentrate very hard, while foggily conscious, to learn anything at all. This caused me to hate interruptions, which I despise to this day. When I am working, I still concentrate so hard on a project that I have great difficulty hearing someone speaking to me. This probably helped complicate life with my teachers and still does when people think I'm ignoring them.

During this time, my parents continued their efforts to help me get control of my seizures. From November through December there are reports of three visits to a hospital in San

Francisco, California. The following January a doctor in Salt Lake City gave a consultation, neurological examination and report covering May to date. This report detailed many changes of medications, combinations, strengths and schedules and proposed additional changes as seizure patterns indicated. In February and March this same doctor gave follow up consultations, in which he further reviewed my physiological situation, performed neurological examinations and made more drug suggestions. He also mentioned that I was attending kindergarten and getting along well despite ten to thirty seizures daily.

As a young girl I asked, if God loved me so much, why He was allowing these problems to happen to me. It was much later that my husband showed me II Corinthians I: 1-4 in the Bible. This says we are comforted by God in our troubles, so we can comfort those in trouble with the comfort we have received from Him. These verses provide a sense of meaning and usefulness to my many problems and are comforting to me when I remember them.

FORT HUACHUCA, ARIZONA

The last medical report was from Fort Douglas, Utah before Dad was transferred to Fort Huachuca, Arizona in the first week of August. Preschool, kindergarten and first grade were all severely influenced by the large number of petit mal seizures I was having in class. Irritability, dullness and other side effects from the medications also were problems for me. They affected the rest of the class, especially my irritability. Never-the-less the medical record says that, although behind in educational level, I was doing reasonably well under the circumstances. The doctors probably were making this judgment based on their observations during my short visits with them and my parents' perhaps optimistic statements.

The records show this came to a screeching halt while I was in second grade in autumn. Statements from school, in doctors' consultation reviews and medical file notes indicate that I was irritable and uncooperative. During this time the changing medicines and medication schedules may have been particularly troubling to me. Each change tended to produce uncomfortable and difficult side effects. Also irritability is a side effect of several of the medications, happening more with some meds, than others. Additionally, I was old enough to think it unfair that I was the only child I knew of, to have these problems. My memories are of the same continuing problems I was having all along. Because of the severity of the problems, the teacher recommended a special class.

Her suggestion was approved and I was placed in a special class in October. Gradually the special class seems to have helped me get a more positive attitude and accomplish more. This included reading at second grade level although <u>not</u> with good comprehension. In June, the special education teacher recommended another year of special education. She said she believed this could enable me to return to a regular class room. Interestingly, despite all my physical problems, I had caught up in reading and was making steady progress in other areas. She pointed out that, "I might be a slow learner," perhaps because of my reading comprehension [input] problem. In looking back, this seems to be a reasonable interpretation. Unfortunately it generally seems to have been interpreted as an indication of a limited <u>overall</u> intelligence.

This compares with many of my doctors who generally said that my relative slowness probably should be attributed to, perhaps controllable, physiological problems. Maybe they had a better understanding of how deeply these problems could affect the patient's life. I suspect that it was easier for teachers to blame slow learning on a lack of <u>overall</u> intelligence, than consider that teaching quality and teaching effort might influence learning speed. But I recognize that I presented an extraordinary teaching challenge. With my seizures, medical side effects, other illnesses and related absences, it must have been difficult to recognize a good ability to manipulate information.

When I was seven or eight years old I wanted desperately to ride a bicycle like the rest of my friends. Because of the seizures I was forbidden to ride and my parents wouldn't buy me a bicycle. So, I quietly borrowed my girl friend's and, in time, became a good rider. Finally, Mom recognized that I was riding anyway, and persuaded Dad to buy a bicycle. I was proud of my riding ability and told my folks that I would join the circus where bicycling, while having seizures, would earn me lots of money. Riding a bicycle made me feel more grown up and accomplished.

Shopping with Mom also made me feel more mature. With four active children, Mom had a tough time keeping us corralled while shopping. I was eight years old; Johan, three, Mike, two and Phil, fifteen months. Rather than chase my brothers around the store, Mom hooked leashes to their belts and kept them in tow. I was old enough and obedient enough that I was unleashed. At times this arrangement drew a reaction from other shoppers. Sometimes it was admiration for Mom's unusual idea. Others it was anger at her supposed cruelty to her children. But Mom didn't care how they felt. It was simply a useful way to keep reasonable control of her children without hurting them and is a nice example of Mom's inventive ideas.

Not all my misadventures were fun and games. One time I took the bus home from school and slept past my regular stop. When I got off, I was lost and wandered around until, finding a church, I went inside. There I told the priest that I was lost. He said, "Well, now you are found." After requesting my phone number; he called my parents to come get me. I was tired; so he gave me a pillow and blanket and let me to sleep on a pew until Dad arrived to take me home.

In December Special Education arranged for a university rehabilitation unit to administer a children's intelligence test. A letter from special education says I was upset by the test situation and would not do the performance scale. Mom told me that this involved putting various shaped and colored blocks in their corresponding holes. She suggested that I was interested more in the shapes, textures and colors of the blocks than in putting them in holes. Also, I may have thought that this was a test for babies while I was in the second grade. Having people underrate me has been a problem all my life and I still dislike it intensely. I scored a verbal IQ of seventy one. The testing psychologist said my emotional reaction to the test situation could have influenced the reliability and validity of the test results. He said I should be retested with about a year's time lag. Despite the test administrator's clear indication of the questionable usefulness of this test result, it has negatively influenced my life with teachers and even my Dad. My test score would normally indicate extremely limited mental ability. The assumption that it was an accurate measurement of my <u>overall</u> intelligence has been proven hugely wrong by what I have achieved.

Unfortunately, the lack of validity of the test result because the test was not completed does not appear to have been properly appreciated. Also, my ability to use information I had absorbed was largely hidden by the overwhelming problems of the seizures and the medicines' dulling effects. The teachers' dependence on the simple test result, reading comprehension difficulties and the statement that I might be a slow learner appear to have worked together to establish reliance on the test score, rather than permit considering other possible interpretations. For whatever reasons, many educational professionals seemed to accept the idea that my <u>overall</u> intelligence was severely limited. Those who accepted this may have reduced trying to teach me as they believed such efforts to be a waste of time.

These unfortunate beliefs and the problem of catching up after the seizures were more under control appear to be the main reasons for still suggesting I be institutionalized. I was socially promoted (without the required learning) for most of the severe seizure years. It made catching up particularly difficult. There were a few teachers who, looked past the IQ test results and my other problems. They saw a person worth helping develop and made special efforts to teach me. This was very helpful and they are deeply appreciated. I still have holes in my bag of knowledge, which it would useful to have closed. For example, I am very poor at fractions and can't read a regular ruler or thermometer. I am able to work around fraction problems by using percentages and ruler problems by asking for help. It is less troubling than you might think, because, early in life, I learned to compensate. Compensating for problems, seeking alternative methods, is a way to manage information, and is a generally recognized sign of intelligence. The habit of looking for other ways to solve life's problems is second nature to me and is very useful in my work today. You rarely recognize the up side of trouble, while in the midst of it.

Note: By now you may have noticed how often I have pointed out that I was intelligent and that the dullness was caused by external factors. This is because the assumed lack of <u>overall</u> intelligence was a constant issue everywhere in my daily life. It was so, even in my home, where Dad believed it. I couldn't fight it successfully in everyone and, not always, in myself. With all of the old statements of my mental limitations to haunt me, I'm still working on it. Thank God, that Mom almost always believed in me, although, even she, wasn't able to hold out against every statement of the educators. My husband and I have been considering the probability that I have some sort of input problem. Probably the biggest barrier to recognition of my overall intelligence has been input. The input difficulty, complications of epilepsy and reactions to heavy medication made finding a reasonable degree of intelligence extremely tough. It required strong interest and persistence. The idea, of an input problem comes first from my personal observations of continuing difficulty in absorbing what I read. It has been strengthened by reading my medical history for the writing of this book. My husband and I plan to have testing done to establish the exact element(s) of the problem and to find what remedies may be available.

The record isn't clear and I don't remember, if I remained in special education at the start of the school year. Its continuation had been recommended by the special education teacher. She made a report to a neurological institute in Arizona about my physical history and accomplishments while in her class. In it she remarked that Dad found it difficult to have me in special class. It appears that he was unable to accept, what he believed to be the shame of it. He was unsuccessful in resisting special class for the last part of second grade. But even if he had to tolerate it for third grade, beginning the new school year he found a way to overcome what he considered to be a problem.

SECOND GERMAN PERIOD

We transferred to a German duty station late in December or early January and I was assigned to a regular class. On January nineteenth there was a psychological evaluation to help establish school placement. Our first quarters were at the same Vogelweh Army Base in Heidelberg. We soon moved to off base housing in Kaiserslautern to be nearer Dad's work assignment. The medical record of places I was seen by doctors suggests that we may have lived in several towns and villages during Dad's second tour in Germany. I remember the names Erlenbach, Heidelberg, Kaiserslautern, Karlsruhe, Landstuhl, Mannheim and Vogelweh. So far, the best I have been able to figure is the following: Vogelweh was the name of the US Army Base where we were first quartered in Heidelberg; Landstuhl, a suburb of Kaiserslautern is where a large US Army Hospital is located; we appear to have moved either to Kaiserslautern or to Landstuhl from base quarters in Vogelweh. We also may have lived in Erlenbach, Karlsruhe and Mannheim or perhaps, only visited there. Unfortunately, all I remember is living on base at Vogelweh and off base at Kaiserslautern (Landstuhl).

Education was not the only thing in my life and in February, despite the seizures, I managed to get into my own foolishness. This happened in Vogelweh on the school playground during recess. One of my school mates challenged me to cross what we called monkey bars. These are overhead ladder like devices, which children swing across one hand hold at a time. I took up his challenge and, part way across, looked down and let go. Upon landing, I sprained my left ankle. Dad came to school and took me to the hospital, where they installed a soft cast. The next day the same boy said I couldn't cross it because I had the cast on. My reaction was, "OH YEAH? Watch me." I started on the monkey bars, went part way across, looked down and let go again! This time I sprained my right ankle and bruised my back. Dad was not too happy about having to take me to the hospital again. He said, "Do that again and I'll break both your legs."

A few weeks later I waited a long time on an especially cold morning for a school bus that never came. My fingertips became painful and turned blue. I developed frostbite in all of them, which turned into gangrene. By the middle of May I was diagnosed as having Raynauds Phenomenon. This limits the flow of blood to the extremities; fingers, toes, ears and nose. The Raynauds attack was so severe that when I picked scabs off my finger tips I could see the bones. I couldn't tie my shoes, brush my hair, write or do many other normal activities. Doctors told my parents, that with the severity of the gangrene, there were only two choices for treatment. One was surgery, on the sympathetic nerve in the upper back, which controls blood circulation and is called a sympathectomy. The surgery might improve circulation to my fingers. The other was amputation of the fingers. My parents chose the sympathectomy, cutting of the sympathetic nerve next to my upper spine after removing a rib.

Fortunately, the nearest Army doctor who dealt with this surgery was at the nearby Landstuhl, Germany United States Army Hospital, where the operation was performed. I was admitted to pediatrics on May twentieth. They transferred me to neurology for drug adjustments to rule out the possibility that the pain and blueness might be a drug reaction. With no indication of that, they transferred me to surgery. The hospitalization was from May to July. Thinking the length of time was punishment, I begged Mom to please take me home. I promised to be good and not get into trouble without success. The food tasted awful and I refused to eat resulting in weight loss. Food brought from home was soon allowed.

The doctor ordered a series of tests, some of which were very uncomfortable. The most frightening was called a ganglia block. As I understood it, this required placing a needle in each side of my throat and pushing them in to have the needle points meet. When I overheard the nurses talking about it before the test, I ran out of the room and down the hall trying to get away. Soon I had nurses, orderlies and my parents chasing me. While running, I looked back and saw them all chasing me. It seemed funny and I started giggling. The more I giggled, the slower I ran and they soon caught me. The test was as difficult as they said.

The sympathectomy which involves cutting of the sympathetic nerve on the side of the spine was performed on one side of my back. Then there was a period of waiting to see if the circulation results were positive with signs of circulation returning to my fingers. They were and the doctor reported to my parents that I was fortunate because he only had to do a unilateral sympathectomy. He was surprised that with the severity of my case he didn't need to cut the nerve on both sides, producing more serious side effects. Also, he told them Raynauds usually happens to people forty to sixty years old. At nine years old, I was setting a record for having a sympathectomy and my story would be in the medical literature.

I was impressed with the fame this would bring me! But more importantly, I would have another claim to fame, the stitches in my back. Soon after the operation, in preparation for school, I found one of Mom's mirrors. I used it with the bathroom mirror to count the stitches. I would be able to report their number to my classmates and maybe even show them how neat the stitches were.

I didn't fully know the side effects of my operation, but would soon find out. The first thing I noticed was a droopy left eye lid. It drooped badly at first, but was less noticeable as time passed. Also my left eye's iris became lighter and the pupil smaller than my right eye's. Most serious was the inability to perspire on my left side. This meant that now, my body had only half a cooling system. But one half is much better than the complete loss of bodily cooling that cutting both sides would have produced. Unfortunately, I would always have to be very careful about over exertion, hot rooms and summer heat. In fact, all extremes of temperature would be dangerous because Raynauds can recur from exposure to cold.

My overheating shows immediately, by producing redness on the perspiring side, along with no color on the other side. This bothered me when people asked about it. Mom said I could tell them by I was half Indian. If I wanted to, I could explain later. While this advice was helpful it could not rid me of the feeling of shame about the way I looked. I sometimes felt like a stranger in my own home and even more so, when outside with people.

This time in Germany was very eventful and has provided me with many memories, some fond and some not so. When we moved off base to Kaiserslautern, we rented the second and third floors of a German family home, while they lived on the first floor. It was located up a hill. Upon opening the upper part of the kitchen Dutch door in the back of the house, we could look out over the valley. In season, we could see cows grazing in the meadow with trees in the background. It was especially beautiful in winter, with a blanket of snow covering everything.

One of my favorite memories is of Mom with arms outstretched to welcome us home. It was a cold winter day when my brothers and I were trudging up the hill from school. The sun was shining brightly on the fresh snow, and Mom was kneeling in it in the front of the house, with outstretched arms, We all ran to meet her and wound up in one big hug in her arms. I felt so loved.

Winter was when going up the hill to the house was most difficult because of ice. The back part of the property was much steeper than the front, but was a shortcut from the school in town. One icy winter day I took the short cut, although afraid to go up the back side because of the steep icy ground and rocks. My friends thought that going around would be too far, and unnecessary. They insisted that I try climbing, which I did, slipping and sliding. Finally, with them pushing, we made it to where I could reach the hand Mom was holding out to pull me the rest of the way. This may feel especially meaningful to me, because I usually felt unlovable. Mom was the only one who would tell me she loved me, encourage me and give a final hand up when I needed it.

One day all of us, except two year old Phil, went outside for some reason and left the house key in the door on the inside. Somehow Phil managed to lock the door. The landlord family was away and we were stuck outside unable to open the door. We all tried to persuade Phil to unlock the door, even Dad. All

Phil did was laugh and run from window to window to look at us. Finally, Dad got a ladder from the neighbors next door, and climbed up to a second floor window. He managed to get in and a minor emergency was solved.

About six months after my operation, Mom gave birth to a beautiful little girl, who she named Danielle. I was very excited because I had waited for a sister for a long time. I wanted a sister to go with my three brothers and eagerly looked forward to helping take care of her. My joy over this didn't last long because she died in her crib one night only a little over two weeks later. They said it was sudden instant crib death. I told Mom Danielle was so beautiful that I was the one who should have died. I felt that way, because I believed the operation had made me ugly and with my problems, I was too much trouble to everyone.

My brother Mike was born tongue tied and couldn't pronounce my name so he called me Shurshur. With his tongue problem, talking was so hard that he practically gave up trying. In his angry frustration he sometimes bit people. Being tongue tied gave him great difficulty in school, especially in Kaiserslautern, with a new language and demanding teacher. One day he became so frustrated and angry that he kicked the teacher on her shin and was suspended from school. Mom and Dad had to assure her this wouldn't happen again before she would allow Mike back in class. After this incident, Mom took Mike to a doctor to see what could be done about his tongue. He said the tissue under Mike's tongue was too tight, which prevented enough tongue movement to speak properly. He recommended cutting some of it, and my folks had him perform the operation. After this and with a little practice, we could hardly get Mike to stop talking. With the new freedom to speak, his bursts of anger disappeared and he never bit anyone again.

After Danielle's death, with Mike's problems and my continuing medical difficulties, Mom had a bad case of depression. She cried all the time and had trouble, even getting out of bed. Dad decided to get a maid to help around the house. The maid seemed alright but after a while, Mom noticed some of her lingerie and jewelry seemed to be missing. She didn't think much about it, deciding they would turn up. Before they did, the police came to our door and hauled the maid away. We learned that she was a thief and some of Mom's things, found in the maid's home, were returned. The police also told us she was a prostitute. This caused Mom to question me about the one time she had sent me to town with the maid. I told her that we had gone past some naked women sitting on window sills. Mom wondered what I might have caught. Immediately, she took me to the hospital for tests to make sure I hadn't somehow caught some disease from the maid. Suddenly, Mom decided we could manage without a maid.

My girl friends and I played a game which we called German jump rope. It used an elastic band instead of regular rope. My friend, Dora, and I wanted to play it, but there was a problem. We didn't have enough money to buy the game from the store. We decided to make our own elastic band cost free. Each of us went home and took the elastic waist bands out of our mother's underpants. We knotted the elastic bands together to make our German jump rope. Our mothers were mystified at first about why their underpants wouldn't stay up. They decided to question us about it. Before questioning me, Mom demonstrated the problem by trying on the underpants in front of me. She asked if I had any idea why it wouldn't stay up and I told her what we had done. I explained that it was an effort to save money. Mom said that she would have to replace the underwear. She said this would be even more expensive than the game. After promising never to do that again, I received some minor punishment.

The German schools were very strict and used a stern disciplinary style of teaching. Teachers were allowed to paddle students. Dora was having a problem keeping up with the class in math. The teacher struck her on the head, causing a concussion. Because of the immense respect given to teachers in Germany at that time, her parents did nothing about the teacher's brutal punishment. But my parents would not ignore the cruelty of what he had done, especially since it could happen to us as well. They protested to the school authorities and had her teacher dismissed.

I still remember many wonderful German foods. For example, our whole family loved the taste of their breads. They were heavy and course in texture, but much more flavorful than breads generally available in chain stores in America. Kaiserslautern's local bakery had a bicycle bread delivery man. He got bread from the oven first thing in the morning and started his delivery. We especially enjoyed those fresh hot breads and made sure to catch the delivery man as he came to the door, to get the hot bread which seemed extra delicious. Perhaps this was because the dense dough was a little softer. But another reason was the wonderful aroma, which filled the whole kitchen.

Another favorite of mine was the German corn fritter. The landlord's wife made them and the first time I saw her set out the ingredients there were some onions. I hated onions and told her I wouldn't eat the fritters. She fibbed, telling me she wouldn't use the onions. However, she told Mom not to worry because the onions would be chopped so small that I would never know they were there. I liked the fritters so much that I gobbled eight or nine of them. Even now, when I see German friends, I ask them to make some for me. It wasn't until later that I found out they contained onions.

I suppose that one of the two or three foods most typically recognized as German food is sauerkraut. I don't remember liking it, but in Kaiserslautern, I learned to despise it. When Mom was going to cook sauerkraut, my responsibility, as the oldest child, was to go to the grocery and purchase it. The grocer took kraut from the barrel, weighed it, wrapped it in newspaper, and I carried it home. Part way home the juice leaked through the newspaper all over me. I hated the smell and still do.

Another time I had difficulty eating German food was when the landlord's wife served us a rabbit dinner. They had purchased three rabbits to grow for food. We assumed that they were to be pets and named them after my brothers, Johan, Mike and Phil. We fed and watered them and enjoyed watching their actions as they grew. Imagine our shock to discover that they were going to be slaughtered and served for dinner. None of us kids were able to eat rabbit that day.

I became familiar with the German beer halls. Perhaps, because at ten, I was five years older than Johan, my oldest brother, Dad occasionally to took me along when he went out drinking. This was very important to me because it was something we could do together. I would sit on the bar stool, order a non-alcoholic Shirley Temple and feel very grown up. I mimicked Dad's language in reordering saying, "hit me again" and tried to make him proud of me.

Sometimes, Dad asked me to pick up a six pack of beer for him. One hot summer day I was on the way home with Dad's beer and decided that God wouldn't want me to be thirsty. So I opened a can and drank it. I felt much better and walked further. But I got thirsty again and drank another one. By the time I got home

I had opened another, and was feeling no pain. I told Mom I was tired; and wanted to go to bed. Dad was upset about the missing beer, but it didn't bother me much. Mom told him that trying to correct me, right then, would be a waste of time. So, I seemed to get through this alright. But the next morning the situation had changed. I had a terrible headache and begged Mom to let me stay home from school because I was sick. She made me go to school anyway, and I never made that mistake again!!

One day while we were visiting the neighbors next door, Dad decided to teach me how to stand on my head. I tried to follow his instructions several times without much success and he decided to demonstrate. He managed to get up alright but had trouble maintaining his balance. He started to tilt and kept on going. He landed with feet through the glass front of the neighbor's china closet. The closet was knocked over and had other damages beside the glass front. Some of the broken china seemed to be heirlooms and must have been valuable. The neighbors were gracious, but Mom was furious and let Dad know it when we got home.

Dad, with his German heritage, loved to play lord of the manor, but he had married an awfully lot of woman to be able to pull it off successfully. Mom was a beautiful woman with a lot of pride, although never aloof. But she was not one to let her husband, or anyone else, walk all over her. With her quick wit and sharp tongue, she easily beat Dad in arguments. She was very talented, bright and athletic and could be quite competitive. She played a mean game of table tennis and usually beat Dad. He had a hard time accepting that she could beat him at anything and hated losing to her at table tennis. She also managed to demonstrate her abilities and competitiveness in other ways. In time, a German driver's license was required to drive on the public roads in Germany. Dad figured he had a U S license and didn't study much for the driving test, which he took and failed twice. Mom studied hard, took it once and passed. He hated having to be driven to work by his wife.

In July, I was seen at Landstuhl U. S. Army Hospital which gave this abbreviated report: "6-8 episodes of tonsillitis in past year, causing loss of 41 school days this year. Chronic tonsillitis-Rx-Sched for T & A." Another hospital report in August gave a short medical summary of the year. It reviewed my tonsillectomy/adenoidectomy and some suturing for hemorrhaging after the operations. Finally I had received the operations which, hopefully, would stop my chronic throat infections.

The October neurology report mentions, "Recent tests in school showed a verbal IQ of 68 & performance of 48. Special class recommended." "Requested testing to determine specific defect." "Appointment made for October 27." "Father cancelled 5 days before the appointment because of imminent transfer to CONUS and stated his preference for the testing to be done there." It referred to a psychiatrist at Fort Gordon, Georgia and giving a date in October mentioned "No seizures since May, '66" and advised hand carrying, "health folder to CONUS. No testing was done. I believe Dad didn't deliver the testing recommendation to Fort Gordon because he wanted to look good and was ashamed of what testing might show.

Note: I still don't know the exact nature of the problem the neurology report referred to, in calling for testing to discover the "specific defect." As I mentioned earlier, my husband has suggested that I finally get the testing necessary to find out. We believe that there is an input problem. This is because I am still a slow reader and have to reread to get satisfactory comprehension. However, I have learned an enormous amount of computer software and am very successful at manipulating it. Furthermore,

I have been the administrative assistant to the internationally known leader of a major world renowned research laboratory with a staff of sixty scientists. My responsibilities varied widely and required reprioritizing with the ebb and flow of assignments. This went reasonably smoothly which convinces me that adjusting known information to changing requirements is not a problem. My apparent strength in manipulating known information has largely compensated for the shortage in entry ability. We plan to find out what steps can be taken to improve information entry and act accordingly.

FORT GORDON, GEORGIA

There were a number of medical reports during the five year period at Fort Gordon in Georgia. They list the return of petit mal and grand mal seizures with various degrees of successful control, and were accompanied by the previous problems of skin rashes and irritability. I continued to have sore throats, severe nose bleeds, upper respiratory infections, headaches, etc. Several of these episodes were bad enough to put me in the hospital for periods ranging from over night to a week or more. However, though inconsistent, the general trend was one of improving seizure control and less drug affect on mental alertness.

About this time, I remember Dad telling Mom, "She acts like she is living in a dream world." After all, I had been through: I didn't appreciate Dad's comment even though he was probably right. How would he know what I was feeling? I was always tired from all the medication, up to thirteen and a half doses daily. Finally one day, Mom told the doctor how tired I was. He said that I would never be completely off epileptic medicine, but suggested taking me off one of them. At this time, I was taking Zarontin, Mysoline, and Dilantin three times daily. For starters he recommended reducing the Zarontin, a little each week until I was off of it. When I was completely off Zarontin, I was more alert and felt wonderful. Family, friends & associates began to notice a big difference in me. I remember saying, "Thank you GOD, thank you GOD for my miracle." No one without epilepsy will ever know what life felt like during those early years. My seizures didn't stop immediately, but gradually, as the dosage was corrected and brought nearly complete seizure control. I didn't have even a petit mal seizure in twenty five years until late in twenty eleven.

With all the problems I had been having, Mom found it difficult to say no to me, even though she probably should have more often. For example, if we went shopping for a dress for a special occasion, she sometimes gave me a choice between two dresses we both liked. I always wanted both and had trouble choosing. Even though it might strain her budget, she occasionally purchased both. Looking back over the years for the preparation for this book, I've come to the conclusion that I was somewhat spoiled.

Mom liked music although she had a poor singing voice. She wanted me to have training in music and the arts and sent me to tap dancing school. I was so poorly coordinated that it became obvious this would never work. (Years later, a doctor told me that Dilantin had been damaging the nerve functions to my large muscles, and I was fortunate to have good motor function in my hands to use for earning a living). She also enrolled me in piano lessons which worked much better. I gradually became skilled enough that, occasionally, I was allowed to play the piano and organ during church functions. These were not without their mishaps, such as when the priest expected me to play an introduction, and then play the entire piece as he would march down the aisle. I forgot and instead, started on the whole piece, which made him wait until it was complete and I could start over.

My brothers also took music lessons and became good with their instruments. Johan chose the accordion, which had belonged to Mom's Dad. He played well enough to perform for functions, until he got tired of having his friends tease him about playing a squeeze box. Mike and Phil, as they reached ages when Mom considered it appropriate, also took music lessons. They chose piano and also became competent to at least play for their own enjoyment. Mike was particularly good at listening to something and playing it by ear. He was also an accomplished painter. With his photographic memory, he could see something, and later paint an excellent rendering.

Between the seizures, the social isolation of being the strange child, and Mom's concern for my safety because of epilepsy, I was much protected and naïve about the ways of the world as they trickled down to children. For example, there were words on the walls of the girl's toilet school that I didn't recognize. One day before class, while there was some chit chat going on, I asked the girl next to me what one of those words meant. She didn't get a chance to answer me. The teacher had heard the inappropriate word. She promptly took me aside to an empty room, where she explained the word's meaning. Then she sent me to the principal's office, where he called me down for having used that word. Neither teacher nor principal paid much attention to what I had to say. Mom was called and, upon arriving, asked me what had happened. I told her that I had seen a word on the toilet wall and was asking the girl at the next desk what it meant. Upon hearing this, Mom asked the principal why he hadn't listened to me. She pointed out that we didn't use this word at our house. In addition, Mom scolded the teacher for telling me about a subject that she felt was a parent's responsibility to teach.

One day, while on the school bus, one of the girls wouldn't leave me alone. She kept hitting and pushing me. I was tired of it; so when we got off the bus and she still continued, I decided to take action. I took off my glasses (they cost a lot of money for Mom and Dad) and grabbed her hair. Then I twisted her all the way around and gave her a black eye. She didn't mess with me again after that, and I felt much better. I hadn't learned how to deal with frustration or anger very well. Although, I have improved I am still learning to handle anger at over fifty five years old.

Fewer seizures seem to have meant more mischief for me to get into and, as the oldest, I usually was the ring leader. At one Halloween we decided to cut the bottoms out of water filled plastic bags at the last minute to bomb the trick or treaters who came to our door. I can't remember why we weren't out trick or treating. Perhaps we were being punished for some earlier misdeeds. The front door had a window with a screen directly above it. We pushed the screen out which made bombing easy. The timing of the water release was precise so that the tricksters got splashed just as they rang the door bell. Mom was in a different part of the house, and we were the ones charged with handing out the candy. We planned to take turns bombing and answering the door. Our water pranks caused fuss enough to get her attention and she quickly put an end to it.

Mom was a very economical home maker, using her sewing skill and sewing machine to repair clothing. She used Simplicity designs to make dresses for herself and me, and pajamas for the whole family. Also, she dyed her single pair of dress shoes a different color each time she and Dad went out to social affairs so that she would appear to have several pairs of shoes. Her purchases of staples for the house were equally careful. In buying food, Mom usually got cheaper cuts of meat and marinated or otherwise tenderized them. She prepared menus in advance, to know what to buy without wasting produce and other perishables. Mom used mass purchasing and the freezer to take advantage of sale prices and to save time and travel costs. She squeezed every possible benefit out of the money at her disposal and often denied herself in the process. This extended even to the most personal purchases. She even skimped on buying sanitary napkins and would use wadded toilet paper in order to save the napkins for me or to use the savings for purchases, mortgage, etc.

With greater awareness of my surroundings, came an increased consciousness that Dad gave my brothers much more attention than me. The preference for my brothers had started when I was five years old with the birth of Johan. Dad played with the boys and recognized their achievements more. This was especially noticeable when various children's awards were presented. He made a point of attending their events. I can't remember his attending any of my little ceremonies, although he had a number of opportunities. I assumed this was because he was ashamed of me and found his behavior very painful. Many future events established Dad's emphasis on looking good. Looking good was not possible with my seizures, and my reputation as a slow learning child didn't help much. I still believe that he was ashamed of me. However, the fact that fathers often want to have sons to play with, and carry on the family name, may also have been a motive for his preference.

I was not conscious of how the enormous effort Mom made to take care of me, with all my problems, made my brothers feel. It was not until I was in my late thirties and read a book about the affect of major disability on other family members. Suddenly, as though a light was turned on, I recognized that my brothers had been feeling left out and unloved by Mom, The unloved part was particularly sad, because nothing could have been further from the truth. Nevertheless, this misunderstanding persisted and may even still. I have come to believe that part of Dad's extra attention to them, was trying to make up, for the relatively less attention they received from Mom. She had to spend much more time and effort on me, with my many serious medical problems. We were a split family, males on one side, and females on the other, with the problems that produces. In this, I had the advantage over my brothers, because Mom was dependable support, while Dad, with his drinking, was not.

As Dad grew older he developed prematurely white hair at his sideburns. Mom decided to surprise him by dying those sideburns to match the rest of his hair. She bought hair dye and waited for the next evening that Dad passed out from too much whiskey. The wait wasn't long and she set to work with us kids watching. We considered this a wonderful practical joke. When Dad got up in the morning, he didn't seem to notice the change. Later we heard that he had been complimented at work, on how well he looked and had been asked where he had the dying done. When he said his wife did it, some asked if he could get her to dye their hair also. Dad didn't seem to enjoy the joke and let the color grow out, but we thought it was hilarious.

Mom's competitiveness and ability to dominate were on display in a swimming pool incident. My parents bought a fairly large out of ground swimming pool, which Dad assembled in the back yard. He also installed flood lights so that they we could enjoy the pool in the evening. One night after they both had a few drinks and had put us to bed for the night Mom and Dad were fooling around in the pool. There was a lot of giggling going on and, somehow, she got Dad's trunks off. She left the pool with them and Dad was stuck out there without trunks for perhaps half an hour. He was unable to leave the pool because the lights would have exposed him to the neighbors. They had noticed the giggling noises and were peering out the windows to see what was going on. Finally she brought him another drink and his trunks.

At Easter, my brothers decided to reenact the crucifixion. They scavenged some boards and nailed together a cross. Phil, the youngest, would be Jesus. Johan, the oldest, would be a Roman soldier. Mike, the middle son, would be Chief Priest. Just as they were preparing to nail Phil to the cross Mom came running out of the house and stopped it, saying that it was getting too real.

I tend to question things, probably because my nine years of uncontrolled mostly twenty to forty daily epileptic seizures and the heavy narcotics prescribed to control them made understanding so difficult. About the time I was thirteen or so a few teachings of the Catholic Church started to trouble me. For example, infant baptism didn't make sense, because I couldn't see how sprinkling water assured belief in a child too young to understand why it was getting wet. Purgatory was a problem too, since I couldn't find it in the Bible and several priests didn't have satisfying explanations. Being brought up as a Catholic was very structured and I usually felt on automatic redial during a major part of the service. The priest read or repeated standard scripts that the audience had heard many times and they read or said memorized responses in the same automatic way week after week. This seemed boring to me rather than stimulating personal interest and I wanted to check out other churches.

When our black neighbor, invited me to her Baptist church I accepted. This was my first visit to a church with a completely black congregation. The singing was enthusiastic and enjoyable, with singing and dancing so exciting that one time I danced on the pew. The style of service encouraged more participation with people in the audience raising their hands and saying amen to parts of the sermon that touched them deeply. It contrasted with the silent style in our white Catholic Church. Also it didn't present the catholic teaching about infant baptism and purgatory. Wanting to attend every Sunday because the service was enjoyable I persuaded Mom to join me once or twice. She said she liked it but had severe reservations because we were Catholic. My complaints do not mean that I look down on all catholic teaching. Only that since no one fully understands God's ways, I am more comfortable finding other Christian interpretations of parts of the Bible which match my personal understandings.

My interest in the Baptist Church caused a huge ruckus in our family. Mom and Dad objected to my going to a non-Catholic church. Mom pointed out that she and her mother were both Catholics and said that going to a non-Catholic church was forbidden. Dad especially objected to my giving my weekly allowance to a different church. His objections surprised me because he was an atheist. He said his being in real estate sales wouldn't allow him to have me attending a black church. I kept after him to let me go. Finally, he decided that it would be alright for me to attend at night; because people would be less able to see who I was and possibly hurt his home sales. As a result I was allowed to attend occasionally.

About then our church got excited about a visit of the large fat local bishop. I was instructed by my parents to address the bishop, "Good morning your Excellency" and curtsey. Forgetting, I said, "Hi there; how are you?" He said, "Hi there yourself." The ladies had fixed a huge lunch for him and the rest of the guests. Considering his size, I asked him if he was going to leave enough food for everyone! There were a group of sisters, sitting next to the bishop hanging their heads at what I was saying. I also asked if he thought he was fat. He said, "Of course, there will be food for everyone and yes, I am fat. However, I have a hard time pushing away from the table when the food is so good." I was still curious about purgatory and later asked him about that. He said that there was none. This left me feeling relieved that I had an answer that made sense to me but wondering about what I considered to be lying.

About this time Dad's mother came to visit us. Nana, as we called her, had difficulty with modern household equipment. She didn't think about maintenance or read instructions. One day she decided to wash the clothes, and used almost the entire box of soap flakes in one load. I tried to tell her that we had soft water and it didn't need that much, but she paid no attention. We soon had suds on the floor in the laundry room and advancing on the rest of the house. She was angry and blamed the washing machine. Another machine problem involved the Electrolux vacuum cleaner. She kept using it until it wouldn't pick up any more and didn't stop then. As with the washer, she said it was a machine problem. It was so completely plugged that we were unable to clear it, and asked our neighbor, who was talented with machinery for help. He dropped what he was doing and started unplugging the hose, which was tightly jammed. It took quite a while with Nana complaining the whole time about the machine and how slow our neighbor was. Fortunately, Nana didn't remain with us very long.

During this time, we had a dog which Dad named Salesman. Dad taught him a number of tricks, such as fetch, roll over, and play dead. He was good at teaching, although I thought that he strung out the rewards to the point of teasing and abuse. Salesman was the first dog in our family that I considered to be mine. We went on walks and played together. He just loved me for who I was, and had no conditions or expectations. This felt good, especially since after my seizures were under control. I was expected to take on a substantial number of family responsibilities. These ranged from helping Mom with whatever project she had in mind, to watching my brothers and helping Aunt Katie. On the one hand, I liked responsibility, on the other, I resented what I considered an excess of it, as I watched my brothers have very little in the way of duties. Salesman didn't want anything from me except to be loved. He was a good companion and a good listener; I could talk to and play with him without arguments.

When it was time for Nana to go home, Dad decided to give Salesman to her, because she was lonely all by herself, and he would make a good companion. Mom didn't object too much, and I lost my buddy. Salesman was really my dog, and I loved him, so it was hard to give him up. He was about ten to twelve years old when Dad gave him to Nana. Since she had no one else, she grew to love him because of all the love he gave and absorbed. Several years later, when we visited her, he was blind, deaf, had lost his hair and had arthritis. It was truly hard for Nana to put him down but she finally did. Salesman was a great dog.

When Johan was eight years old, he started getting interested in Dad's golf equipment. Dad noticed this several times and told Johan not to touch his golf outfit. One day while Dad was at work, and Mom was in another part of the house, Johan couldn't stand the temptation any longer. He got a golf club and ball and went to the front yard. There he swung the club hard at the ball, which went a few feet without hitting anything. But the swing was hard enough that the club slipped out of his hands. It flew into the double paned picture window, where it stuck. Mom, hearing the crash of glass, called from upstairs asking what the noise was. I replied, "Nothing." She yelled, "That was the loudest nothing I've ever heard" and came running. She looked at the situation and when I started to get the club from the window, she said to leave it there until Dad came home, because he would never believe it. I teased Johan about how Dad was going to punish him severely. Poor Johan was so scared that he was shaking, and I felt ashamed of myself for scaring him. When Dad arrived home he saw the golf club in the broken window immediately. His first words were, "How? How? How"? Dad punished Johan and, life went on at our house.

One of the sports that my brothers and I enjoyed together was baseball. Since we lived in an area with little traffic, we played in the street in front of the house. Once when Johan was pitching and I was at bat, his pitches were hitting the ground before getting to the plate. I told him to move closer, but he was not close enough. He moved closer still, and I was able to hit the ball. This was working well, until I struck the ball solidly, and it hit Johan on the forehead. It knocked him down and momentarily out. A car was coming but I managed to get him out of the street before it became a problem. Johan had a large lump on his head that showed the stitches of the baseball cover. He said that when I hit that ball, all he could see, before being knocked out, was baseball.

We kids rarely had the opportunity to do much with Dad. It was a real treat when we were invited to go crabbing with him. This was particularly so for me since I was excluded from most things he did with the boys. These excursions started early in the morning, before sunrise, to get to the bay early. Crabbing was a major production with chicken necks being aged several days in a bucket to get them nice and stinky and more attractive as bait for the crabs. We baited the crab traps, which we pulled up by cords attached to them. Mom usually didn't come along because her fair skin sunburned very quickly. After we got a good mess of crabs we would head for home with them and Dad would cook them with spices for a crab feast.

Later, when Phil was ten or eleven he found another use for chicken necks. He had become angry with one of the neighbor fathers, who had said something about him, which he believed to be unfair. When Phil heard that the neighbor's family was going to be out of town for the weekend, he decided to get back at him by playing a nasty trick. The houses in our area had individual mail boxes on posts that were at the street. Phil took some of the chicken necks which had been ripening for bait and put them in their empty mail box. Then he locked it with an old unused padlock and threw away the key. It was summer time in Georgia so naturally the necks continued to ripen. By the time they got home, two days later that mail box really stank. They had to cut the lock off the mail box and had no way to establish who did it. Phil was so pleased with himself that he couldn't keep it secret and they eventually found out. They complained to Mom and she punished Phil.

When we went crabbing, Dad would sometimes bring back mussels in a covered bucket. One time he put the bucket in the garage and forgot about it. A couple of weeks later he noticed that the garage had a bad smell. Sometimes garages do smell from the variety of chemicals stored in them, and the smells which can come from a car. He didn't look for the problem right away and the smell got worse. Finally the stench was so bad that he couldn't put the search off any longer, and he started checking the crabbing gear to see if somehow a crab had been left in a trap. Nothing was wrong there, but when he opened the bucket, **WOW!!**

I found arithmetic difficult and my parents hired a tutor to help me with it. I went to his house to work on my arithmetic in the afternoons. He was quite helpful, but as we continued to work on the math problems afternoon he started to massage my back. This continued and gradually became more and more sexually related. I didn't know what to do about it, but it made me feel dirty and I took baths to try to feel clean. Finally, I asked Mom about what he was doing. Mom questioned me closely and told me not to allow myself to be touched like that. She said that this was something to be saved for marriage and I was forbidden to have anything to do with him. Then, she asked if anyone else had done any of those things to me. I told her that a relative had so I didn't see anything wrong at first. She, horrified, gave him a piece of her mind and promised not to leave me alone with him.

Meanwhile, my folks fired the tutor and were trying to find out what could be done. They found a lawyer who listened carefully to them and to me. He said that no charges could be made to stick because of my youth and consciousness problems. The seizures and the medicine I was taking would make it more difficult to get a conviction. Inability to defend myself in this situation was a huge disappointment because rumors that I was having sex with the tutor were flying around the neighborhood and were a tremendous embarrassment to me.

There were times when Dad could no longer stand Mom's superior wit, arguing ability and fierce tirades. Usually he charged out of the room or left the house to cool down. But sometimes he used physical violence to gain dominance. Mom told me of one time when they were walking by the base trash dump and were having a loud and very public argument. Dad probably had a few drinks, which usually brought out the worst in him. Something she said infuriated him, and he shoved her into the trash. She came out swinging and caught him right on the nose, which started to bleed. The base commander, who happened to be walking by, saw it and told Dad, "We don't push our wives into the trash." Then he said to Mom, "We should have you in the Army."

When Dad completed twenty years of military service, he decided to leave the Army and was discharged as a Major, his final rank. The Army had a ceremony to honor him and other officers. There was a band, marching and awards. At the ceremony we kids felt proud of Dad and decided to join the parade. As the marching troop passed by we were at the end of it, marching right along. Now Dad would have to get another career because the monthly retirement income of about four hundred dollars was too little to meet our family's needs.

AUGUSTA, GEORGIA

Dad got his first job out of the service teaching at a nearby college but it didn't pay well enough to meet the family's needs. In order to increase the family income Dad started part time to sell products of a multilevel distributorship and recruit others into it so as to get commissions on their sales. It was 'gung ho' at first with the whole family involved. I had no interest in the recruiting of other distributors to work in our organization but enjoyed selling the products. To become profitable a distributorship seems to require talent for both recruiting and sales. It demands the self discipline needed for any outside commission sales work. Also, considerable organizational ability is necessary to juggle recruiting, sales, product ordering, inventory and delivery in the right mixture of activity. Furthermore, a high level of optimism needs to be maintained by the distributor, the immediate members of family sales staff, and the recruited people. With my physical problems, three other children and a house to take care of, Mom didn't have the time or energy to take on much of this additional activity. Dad, with his self doubts, couldn't maintain the optimism and didn't have the structure of the military to make up for his lack of personal self discipline and responsibility. As the result our family's distributorship period was relatively short.

One of the props used by distributors to impress recruits with the success possible was displaying their own motor homes for vacations. Dad had seen one owned by a distributor up the distributor line and caught the motor home fever. He decided that we would rent one for a week's vacation. Off we went, and while we were on the road, Mom and I used the toilet on board. After a few minutes water was running out of the toilet across the floor. I told Dad and he pulled to the side of the road as soon as he could. Somehow, Mom and I had plugged the commode with toilet paper and the flushing mechanism had kept flowing. Dad managed to shut off the flow and unplug the paper jam. After we mopped up the floor, we resumed our trip. But this ended his interest in motor homes.

One weekend, during a trip in the country, Mike saw some cows in a field. Some were brown and some white. He told us that he had figured out where chocolate milk comes from. Mike said that white cows give white milk and brown cows give brown milk. He said that to get it out, you pump the tail up and down. I thought that's original, but the cow wouldn't be too cooperative with that, and chuckled at Mike's logic

During this period, Mike and I started selling Christmas cards to make ourselves some extra money. Mike, very bold, would knock at any door and start his sales pitch. He said things like, "Look at the richness of the color," and "Feel the quality of the paper." He was so cute that he sold quite a few boxes of cards. I was more timid and wouldn't knock where it said no sales allowed. But I sold my share of cards and particularly remember one neighbor who had a no sales sign. I always avoided his house. But his curiosity got the best of him and he had to find out what I was selling. He came out, invited me in and bought several boxes of cards. I learned that in sales, no doesn't always mean no.

After teaching at the nearby college, Dad started selling several styles of prefabricated homes either already in place or to be built on real estate owned by a local developer. As soon as Dad arrived from work we children would ask him if he sold any houses today. It takes a while to establish yourself in real estate sales and the answer usually was no. Mom took us aside and told us that we must stop asking about sales all the time. She said it's hard enough not making sales, without having to report no sales to your children almost every day.

With his technical knowledge, he sometimes designed the prefabricated housing elements into homes to meet customer desires. Because of this, we would occasionally receive phone calls asking about details of housing plans. They asked questions such as dimensions of a specific room, or distance of a door from a particular wall. I learned to answer the simple questions and was glad to be able to help. I received a call from a man asking details about one of the standard houses on a certain home site. When I finished the description, answered his questions and quoted the established price he said that he wanted to buy. I was excited and told Dad as soon as I saw him. He said, "That's impossible. "Nobody buys a house without looking at it." But when Dad phoned the caller, he confirmed his decision and Dad had another sale.

During this time, possibly at Christmas, I was given my first camera. It was a Polaroid Land camera, the first camera so far as I know, to print the pictures without requiring the film to go through an entirely separate development process. I was very excited with my new toy and went about taking pictures of the neighborhood. I especially enjoyed scenes with clouds and blue sky as background. This was so much fun for me that Mom rationed me to one pack of film per week, when my new hobby started to get too expensive for Mom's budget.

After a period of limited home sales, Dad decided he might do better in Atlanta. He looked in the Atlanta newspapers for advertisements for real estate salesmen and obtained an interview. The whole family went along on the interview as a family excursion. Unfortunately, the interview did not result in a job, and we returned home.

During this time, Mom's tiny but feisty Aunt Katie came to live with us. With limited space in the house, she was installed in the living room. Because of her advanced age and the distance to the bathroom, she had her own portable toilet next to her bed. Dad was still selling prefabricated homes and would occasionally bring a prospective buyer home to design the prefabricated units into a house to fit the buyer's wishes. As you may imagine, the picture of Aunt Katie's bed and toilet in the living room didn't help impress the buyer with the competence of the designer/salesman or the company. So Aunt Katie was soon moved next door into her own trailer, and I was assigned to help her because of her frailty and advanced age.

With all of us children, more able to help around the house and household income still too low, Mom decided to try and help by getting a job. She found one at an insurance company in Augusta and worked there until we moved from town. After starting as a receptionist, she progressed gradually to supervisor and then accounting manager. Mom was proud of receiving a paycheck and being able to help Dad with the finances. But that was not enough for Dad. He said she was just making peanuts, although those peanuts paid the monthly mortgage, food, bills and, of course, his booze when he made no sales.

After several years in sales, Dad returned to the steady income of teaching. This time it was at a vocational high school in nearby South Carolina although we continued to live in Augusta. He was knowledgeable enough that several publishing houses contacted him to write books. Dad became quite popular with the students, who told me how lucky I was, to have him for a father. I found this surprising because he seemed to be a different person at home. Perhaps I should have remembered that he always felt comfortable with the soldiers under his direction, although rarely with officers above him. Teaching seemed to be going reasonably well, but it still produced too small a salary to meet our family needs. So Dad continued looking for some way to earn more.

Although it looked alright outside, our house was not well maintained. A number of things needed either preventive maintenance or repair. Mom told Dad that the drain pipe under the kitchen sink was leaking and needed fixing. She asked him to come to the kitchen to show him, and he did. She pointed to the leak but he still didn't see it. So she put her finger on the point of the leak at the bottom of the J shaped trap under the sink drain. Her finger went right through the pipe and the remaining water gushed out. Dad was angry that he had to stop what he was doing and replace the trap immediately. We kids thought Mom's putting her finger through the pipe was funny, although we didn't make a big thing of it in front of already upset Dad.

That year I decided to bake the family's Thanksgiving turkey. I had watched Mom do it over the years and felt that it was my turn now. After all, what could go wrong? I was careful to rinse the bird and made sure to remove any pin feathers. I remembered the right oven temperature, to time the roast according to weight and to baste during roasting. One thing was a little puzzling; the gizzard, heart and neck seemed to be missing. No problem, the bird could be roasted without them. I remembered to start the roast with the bird breast down on a V shaped rack to make it juicy and watched the roasting very carefully. I made sure to turn it over in time to brown the breast. It came out of the oven a beautiful golden brown, and I felt very proud. Mom had prepared the rest of the meal and we all sat down to eat. Dad started to cut the turkey and, part way through, discovered a little something extra, the missing turkey giblets. I was embarrassed, but everyone had a good laugh. I've never forgotten the giblets again.

This period of our lives was troubling with Mom and Dad squabbling much of the time. There was plenty to argue about. The retirement money was not enough to support the family and Dad's drinking. Dad wasn't selling enough to make up the shortage, and the house needed repair. There was enough disagreement that Mom and Dad were sleeping in separate bedrooms. The leak in the roof brought down the ceiling in the master bedroom and Dad moved out of there into the family room. Now that the leak had gotten so bad, Dad fixed it; but it took a while longer to repair the ceiling.

The twenty fifth anniversary of my parents wedding was approaching and we children wanted to make it a special occasion, to help heal the trouble they were having in getting along with one another. We set to work to earn extra money for presents. I chose an expensive hinged silver picture frame for our present and arranged for an anniversary cake to be baked very inexpensively by a neighbor down the street. She loved to bake cakes especially for weddings and anniversaries. It was her passion, and she really enjoyed doing this for people that she knew. Unfortunately, these items cost more than we had earned and I had to beg Dad for an additional twenty dollars.

It had been Mom and Dad's anniversary and I thought Dad should have bought something really pretty for Mom. Instead, he bought an electrical appliance, which did not go over very well with her. One day I saw some attractive nightgowns, slippers and socks in a catalogue that had arrived in the mail. I saved my money and bought her some nightgowns. When they arrived I wrapped them in a box and asked my girlfriend to write on it, "To Mary from Buddy," so they couldn't tell it was my handwriting. Mom was excited and thanked Dad, but he denied buying them. My trying to help Mom and Dad get over their disagreements had made matters worse. Dad questioned us children and, when he found out that I had ordered them, I was in trouble for misrepresenting him.

It was about this time that I had a basic change of heart about Dad. When I was the only child I was very conscious of his love. However, as I got older and had brothers without my disabilities he became more distant. When I was a young girl, I wanted a husband like Dad. As I got older and thought about it I changed my mind. He was abusive to Mom and me and also to my brothers. I didn't recognize their abuse until talking with them years later. Dad told Mom, he didn't want his daughter going for epilepsy counseling. Although he had never attended any of these meetings, he claimed that all they did was cry and hold each others' hands. Neither parent understood why I was angry about being denied counseling, but I needed to talk to people around my age, with similar conditions, so we could compare notes. This didn't happen until I was an adult. It was a shame to wait so long for something that could have been useful much earlier. Counseling was there for people like me and for the people who had to live with them.

One night, when Mom had more than she could bear of the craziness in our family and the constant excess of responsibility, she drank too much and started dozing at the dinner table. I told her she should go to bed (in order to sleep it off). She agreed, but just sat there and dozed off again. After several attempts, I finally talked her into going to bed. But the next thing I knew there was smoke coming from the bedroom. She had fallen asleep with a cigarette in her hand. I doused the mattress with water and checked to see if she was alright. She was unhurt, except for a minor burn on her wrist, which I helped treat with vegetable oil. The mattress had a hole in it and had to be replaced.

We were constantly moving, and I attended at least fourteen schools during the fourteen years it took me to graduate from high school. I believe that Dad was bounced around because he could not get along with his superiors. In the military, they promoted their people or, if they were too much of a nuisance, they transferred them. This did not help in making and keeping friends, going to the same school or having some roots. The frequent change was hard on the whole family. After retiring there from the Army, Dad could not settle down. Perhaps it was the continuing problem of finding a way to earn enough money to pay the bills. We continued moving around after his retirement

Georgia's public schools were going through the struggles of integration and bussing with strong emotions in the students and their parents. To spare us the disruption and confusion which accompanied this social change our parents decided to send us to a Catholic school in nearby South Carolina. Dad was teaching there and could provide transportation. I graduated there from eighth grade at the age of sixteen. Because of my educational difficulties, the educators there recommended vocational training. It was a recommendation which Dad heartily endorsed. Mom believed the educators this time, possibly because they were Catholic.

I was placed in a vocational school in nearby, South Carolina. I had begged Mom to let me attend a regular junior high school, but convincing her of my readiness for regular school was very difficult. I told her that getting credits toward regular school graduation from classes in vocational school would be very slow if not impossible. By the time I would get the credits, I would need to purchase a cane or a wheelchair to get to graduation. Several months after starting the vocational school two of my classmates were raped.

Then Mom accepted my appeals and arranged a transfer to my neighborhood junior high school, in Augusta. It was a feeder school for Butler High and I was able to remain with my friends as I moved up to Butler. Getting a high school diploma was hard work, because I had to make up for the time lost in unrelated classes at the vocational school. I was determined to prove the doctors and educators, wrong; in thinking I couldn't do regular school work. With the help of some really good teaching, doubling up on some courses and summer school, I caught up with friends in my regular class. I wanted desperately to graduate with them but this wouldn't happen because of Dad's decision to move again.

From the time I started learning to print and write I had a continuing problem of very large writing. Over the years, my writing had become smaller, but was still larger than my teachers wanted. On my nineteenth birthday Mom bought a portable typewriter to use for my homework. This was particularly useful because it would help solve my problem of large writing. I had trouble typing in the dim light of my bedroom, and tried using the kitchen table, where there was plenty of light. Dad came home from work, drunk and angry about something. He ordered me to take the typewriter back to my bedroom, but I said I was almost done. He, still drunk and now angrier at not being obeyed immediately, threw the typewriter on the floor.

It broke beyond repair and now, I was furious. Waiting until everyone was asleep I snuck out to the carport, where I slashed two tires on the passenger side of the family car. They were on the side away from the house, and Dad wouldn't notice the flat tires until he tried to drive to work. I knew that Dad would punish me severely when he found them; so I made preparations to be away from home for a while. I rose early the next morning and packed a few clothes in my school bag. When I saw Dad in the morning at breakfast I said nothing about the typewriter. He asked if I wanted a ride to school, but I said I already had a ride with a girl friend. I rushed through breakfast and was well out of the house with my friend before time for Dad to leave for work. I told my friend what was going on, and went home with her after school. I remained until dark and Dad had time to somewhat calm down. When I arrived home, I found out that Dad had been driving around looking for me. He was relieved to see me, but that didn't prevent my being punished, perhaps less severely, than while he was still furious.

Dad decided to teach me to drive our family automobile well enough to pass the South Carolina driving test. I told him that, with my poor coordination, I didn't think I would be able to drive, because of the car's stick shift transmission. Maybe an automatic would have been alright, but not a stick shift. We started training in empty parking lots with my having great difficulty shifting gears, There were grinding noises as I tried to shift and, when I finally got the car in gear, it lurched. Sometimes it stalled but, gradually, I got a little better. Then Dad decided to try traffic. We started out of the parking lot to turn left into the traffic in the street. I was feeling nervous because I didn't think I was ready for traffic, and a left turn across traffic was particularly scary. I was very slow and, with cars coming, we lurched through the intersection. This time Dad was scared too, and he scrunched down in his seat halfway to the floor. Finally he agreed that with my poor coordination I should not attempt to drive a stick shift automobile.

About this time Neil Diamond appeared in concert at the Coliseum in Columbia. I was, and am a fan of his and wanted see him in person. Dad thought I should have an escort to take me to the event. So, I bought tickets for Johan and myself and arranged to stay at a hotel after the concert because it would be too late to catch a bus home. After the concert Johan and I were walking from the Coliseum to the hotel, when Johan said he was thirsty. We decided to get a soda pop. Johan had paid for his, and I was in the cashier's line waiting to pay for mine. Then I noticed several police officers questioning him. Evidently, Johan looked like someone who had robbed the store. An officer asked me if Johan had been with me the entire night and I told him, "Yes." I thought, 'who's the one needing an escort? Here I am speaking for him to keep him from being arrested.' When Mom phoned the next morning to check on us, I couldn't resist telling her of Johan's questioning by the police. My tattling didn't please Johan, but the irony of the situation was too sweet to resist.

COLUMBIA, SOUTH CAROLINA

Dad decided to move again to suburban Columbia, South Carolina where I attended Irmo High School from which I graduated. I would have preferred graduating from Butler High, but couldn't have even that. The ceremony was held at the Columbia Coliseum. I had arranged with a girl friend's family to live with them so that I could graduate with my friends from Butler. I was unable to attend my senior year there, because Dad insisted that I live at our new home. I suspect that Mom had mixed feelings about this and was willing to let Dad be the bad guy who refused to allow me to graduate with my neighborhood friends.

My grandparents made a special trip from Charleston to see the ceremony, and Grandma confided in me that they had never expected me to graduate. I'm sure she meant this as a complement to my persistence, but I made a mental note that, like the rest of the world, they didn't think much of my abilities.

In February I discovered that I was not the only one to have epilepsy in my family. My eleven year old brother, Phil, had a seizure at a tennis court Mom and I ran down and found

Phil being taken to the hospital. Since then, Phil has been on medicines similar to mine.

Mom and Dad were having another argument in our apartment in Columbia and she complained about being manhandled. Dad, nasty as usual when drunk, exploded and said, "I'll show you manhandling." He shoved Mom into the back room, where he beat her. During the beating he broke her ear drum and her ear bled. When he came out of the room I told him, with a kitchen knife in my hand, that if he ever struck Mom again, I'd kill him. Mom never heard with that ear again. Neighbors had heard the noise and called the police. They came to the door, which I answered. They asked everyone questions and asked Mom if she wished to press charges. She said, "No" and they asked Dad if he had settled down enough to remain in the house. He said, "Yes" and, since Mom refused to press charges, they allowed him to stay. But they told him if anything like this happened again, it would mean an automatic ride to the police station.

CHARLESTON, SOUTH CAROLINA

Dad decided that he might make more money in Charleston, South Carolina. So we moved from our apartment in Columbia into a house on Lindberg Street in Charleston. While we children didn't want to relocate, the move had at least one comical moment. Dad had folded and tied the queen sized mattress with cord, in order to fit it around the bend in the hall, on the way to the bedroom. Even with the mattress folded, he was having a struggle moving it. The string, holding the mattress folded, got stuck on a bathroom door. Dad, off balance and with his hands full, asked me to remove the string. I did, and the unfolding mattress sent him flying into the next room on his butt. All that was hurt was his pride, and I couldn't help but laugh.

It was in Charleston that I got my first regular job, as a waitress in a restaurant. My first night at work was on a busy Friday, with white uniformed Navy sailors in town for the weekend. It started out alright, but I had a major waitressing disaster. Part way through supper four handsome young Navy sailors sat down at one of my tables. I took their orders for spaghetti with tomato and mushroom sauce. I was feeling pretty comfortable about having gotten the orders quickly and promptly returned with the spaghetti. Really enthusiastic, I grabbed two plates and tossed them on the table in front of the first two sailors. Without looking, I turned around and served the other two the same way. Then, looking at my customers, I saw an incredible mess. The spaghetti sauce had spilled off all four plates onto the laps of the brilliant white pants of all four sailors, a perfect score. Of course, I offered to pay the cleaning bills and, to my amazement, they didn't raise a fuss and left me a one penny tip. Perhaps, this was because the restaurant owner explained this was my first time waitressing. I was greatly surprised that he didn't fire me and instead taught me to place food down flat and gently, without endangering the customers. Of course, I followed through on my offer replacing all four white pants including tailoring and one shirt. The sailors appreciated my supplying replacement apparel and later I spent a very pleasant day with them as their guest.

I worked there a couple of years until I applied for and obtained a clerical job at a local technical college. A section of the school was devoted to thirty students supported by a U S Government contract. I was the clerk responsible for the details of administration under supervision of an administrator of the school. He let me work with considerable independence, while he was often involved in his work with other units. The contract was completed after I was there seven months and I was laid off along with the other people supported by the contract. I received a nice letter of recommendation, which I still have.

While I was working for the college my boss told me that if I re-used the coffee grounds, I could save money by buying less coffee. I told Dad about this way to save money on coffee and he said he would try it. The next morning, he made coffee with used grounds that he'd dried in the oven and asked if I wanted to try it. I said, "No, you go first." He took a sip and said, "I've been poisoned." It must have had a terrible taste, because he threw both the coffee and the grounds away and made a new batch.

For a while I was the only one in our family having seizures. But one day as I was taking care of my brothers, who were playing in the back yard, sixteen year old Johan started to have a grand mal. Mike and Phil came running to tell me. I remember sitting lightly on him so he wouldn't hurt himself with the convulsions. I was trying to open his mouth so he would breathe. (Please note that the most recent information on dealing with seizures is to keep fingers and other objects out of the seizing person's mouth. The correct thing to do is to make the person as comfortable and safe from bruising and broken bones as possible until the convulsions are over.) In spite of my own seizures I had never seen anyone else have one, and watching Johan have a seizure was very upsetting. My heart felt as though it was pounding in my throat as I was trying to get him to breathe. Finally, he sat up screaming at me, and I just cried and held him. Johan seemed to outgrow his seizures, but when he was taking the seizure medicines his personality changed. The change was to an extremely negative attitude about life and especially toward Mom and me. I believe he hated me to the day he died and held me responsible for most of what happened in our family

Aunt Katie broke her hip and needed help since she was confined to bed. She was moved next door to us in her trailer so that we could look after her. Her dog, a border collie named Mandy, came along with her and was her watch dog, stationed outside for protection. Mandy wanted to please and generally was very obedient. The exceptions were when she was in heat; it was difficult to keep her tied up or on a leash. One time she broke away and disappeared for several days. Then she came back bedraggled and pregnant. She was a fine watchdog, guarding the trailer so that no one could enter unless we said it was OK.

I was assigned to helping Aunt Katie and found her interesting and fun, but demanding. Besides looking out for her safety, I helped Mom prepare her meals and shopped for her groceries, and medicines. As she aged, she required more and more help. One day when I returned from shopping for her groceries, I found her on the floor in a pool of blood. She had fallen and was unable to get up or call loud enough for help. She had lain there for quite a while. I called Mom to come and help me. We lifted Aunt Katie up and onto her bed. Her skin was very fragile and, where she had cut her leg, the skin had been brushed back. We took her to the doctor, and he told us what to do in order to take care of her. After this, my parents moved my bed into the trailer so I could be there to help her

Living with Aunt Katie was a pleasure and relieving to be out of the middle of my parents' conflicts. She loved sweets but was not supposed to eat them. I, occasionally, shared some with her and we enjoyed this secret together. I was paid at the college once a month and, after paying Mom my share of the household upkeep, I squirreled away most of my earnings. My favorite hiding place was under the mattress of my bed, along with other hiding places in my room. Aunt Katie purchased a new bed for me, and I didn't think about the hidden money, until after I arrived at work, on the day of the bed's arrival. In a panic, I phoned Mom to please find and protect my money. She found well over five hundred dollars and asked why I hadn't put it in a bank. I said that with all the bank robberies in the news I didn't trust banks. At her insistence, I opened a bank account.

As Aunt Katie continued with us her frailty became more of a problem. Her failing memory, especially as it applied to remembering medication, was also difficult for us. No one had time to be a constant nurse and she frequently forgot her meds or took them over again. Finally Dad said that either Aunt Katie had to leave, or he would leave. We had a friend who was a nurse in a nursing home, so we arranged for Aunt Katie to live there. She seemed reasonably happy there, partly because they had a piano. She loved to play the piano and liked to play it for me, when I went to visit her. However, there was a fly in the piano ointment. Another patient, having had much more musical training, could play better. She was so good that I especially enjoyed hearing her play. This annoyed Aunt Katie, who was very competitive and wanted my undivided attention. She asked me if I liked her playing better than that old bat's. I didn't dare say, "No." Aunt Katie's stay there was short, as she died just a few months later.

After being laid off from the college, I applied to a Charleston charity and took a job in their clerical pool. I had a variety of duties such as: typing letters and envelopes, stenciling, filing, and answering the phone. Also, I assisted in their functions. This was good for me, working for and with people that I enjoyed. However, one morning after a year or so, I started having a severe pain in my abdomen. I thought perhaps it was the pain of a menstrual period. After working part of the day, I fainted. One of my co-workers brought me home and told my parents what had happened. They immediately took me to the hospital, where the doctor ran a lower GI test. He found nothing, but when he ran the upper GI, he found over 100 gallstones. The next day a surgeon removed my gall bladder, and I was released from the hospital in three or four days. This meant staying home for a couple weeks, not something I wanted to do.

I liked the steady structure that the charity provided. It compared very favorably to the relative chaos of my parents' squabbling and drunkenness at home, which was now extending to my brothers. Johan and Mike had started on alcohol like Dad. They also became nasty when drunk. Another complication of their drinking was driving while under the influence. They were hard on our automobiles and a danger to themselves and others. Fortunately although they caused some accidents they never struck any one with the cars. Phil wasn't a heavy drinker although he used marijuana. Johan, as the oldest of the boys, was looked up to by his brothers. He led them into lots of foolishness and some genuine trouble as the years went by.

Dad was out of work for some time, and as the only one working, I was trying to support six people on a secretary's salary plus his limited retirement. Dad became desperate and, unknown to the rest of us, bought a gun, intending to commit suicide. One day the sound of a gunshot came from the bathroom that was between my bedroom and my parents' bedroom. Mom, my brothers and I thought Dad had tried to take his life. We rushed to him, and he said he was trying to, but that the gun went off while he was raising it and shot a hole in the ceiling. We persuaded him to change his mind about suicide and Mom insisted he get rid of the gun.

In Charleston my brothers started getting high like dad. Johan and Mike got there jollies on booze and Phil started with marijuana. The drinking started in their mid teens, during their high school years, and increased in use, as they grew older and more independent. With Dad drinking heavily for many years, I guess it was a natural progression. I never have gotten into alcohol or other kinds of mind altering drugs. It seems to be a combination of things, possibly the bad experience I had with the beer in Germany when I was picking up Dad's six pack and knowing that alcohol or other recreational drugs would be dangerous with the prescription medicines that I still need daily. Also, I value consciousness too much to want to tamper with it. With all the struggles I had in achieving a reasonably conscious life, free of seizures, altered consciousness didn't hold a lot of appeal. One of the ironies of my brothers' drinking was Dad's anger when they were drunk. He was the prime example of drunkenness in our family.

Now, Mom got drunk too, with the overwhelming stress of all the responsibilities. This occasionally left me as the only sober family member, feeling responsible for carrying on. Phil started following his brothers' leads, about fourteen, growing marijuana plants in the back yard. I remember thinking Phil's plants had pretty leaves, and showing Dad. He asked what was wrong with me for not knowing it was marijuana, and yelled at Phil for growing it. Then he ripped out the plants and told him, "no more."

Johan and Mike got their driver's licenses at the age of seventeen. Careful at first not to drink and drive, they grew careless as time went by. One memorable week Johan's accident with the car had just been repaired and within it Mike crashed it again. Dad phoned the insurance company to tell them about the accident and they said, "We know, we just fixed it." Dad said, "I mean the new one." They insisted the boys be taken off the policy. That ended their driving for a while.

A year or so later, Mom went to a local Charleston hospital with emphysema, to have fluid removed from her lungs. When Mom got home from the hospital, she received a phone bill, which totaled about eight hundred dollars. Johan had developed a crush on a girl who lived in Augusta, and had been constantly on the phone with her. My parents said that Johan would have to pay the phone bill. By this time Johan had shown enough irresponsibility that they didn't trust him to stop making repeated long distance calls. They installed a lock on our old rotary dial phone, so that a key was necessary to use it. Since I had been working steadily for several years and was contributing substantially to the house budget I had my own phone in my bedroom. When Johan discovered the home phone locked, he used my phone in my absence. So I had to get a lock for mine, too.

When Johan was twenty two he moved to Springfield, Virginia, where he got a job as a computer operator from which he soon was discharged. He claimed that they had loaned him money and that, when he couldn't repay it, they fired him. Because he had gotten into Mom's pocketbook without her permission, I didn't believe it was a loan. Before long Phil went to live with Johan in Springfield and also took a course in computer operating. He completed the course, got his certificate, and sought employment as an operator.

About this time Phil met a bright young college graduate named Virginia. Romance developed and Phil moved in with her. When she got a fine offer for a job in southern California, she packed some of their things and flew there. After renting an apartment in Pomona, most of their remaining belongings were shipped. Phil packed up what was left and drove the car the three or four day trip to join her. Once there, he found a job using his computer training.

After Mike graduated from high school he joined the Army and was sent to Fort Knox for basic training. While there, he became very homesick and despaired of being able to complete basic. I remember my parents getting a message from someone in the Army, perhaps the Chaplain, to come encourage him. Maybe he became more used to Army life and made new friends, because when Mom and Dad finally arrived, the sergeant said that Mike had successfully completed basic training. Knowing that Mom and Dad were coming to see him may have helped overcome his depression and contributed to his success. Mom was a positive influence, and Mike would not have wanted to disappoint Dad. He developed a passion for parachuting, which he learned in the Army. His enlistment was for two or three years and to the best of my recollection he received an honorable discharge. After he got out he continued taking parachuting lessons and practiced regularly. He kept a log each time which showed what altitude he jumped from and at what altitude his chute opened. He invited me to go with him and try it. The very thought of it scared me and I refused. He also wanted to learn to fly, which seemed more interesting.

I continued working for the charity until an appealing phone call from my brother Johan about job opportunities in Northern Virginia. I resigned and requested closure of my retirement account. The retirement money along with my savings would help me get started in the new adventure in the Washington, D.C. metro area to find better paying work,

ALEXANDRIA, VIRGINIA

Johan's phone call about the many good jobs and public transportation lured me to Northern Virginia. He said if I wanted to join him at his nice apartment in Alexandria, I was welcome to stay with him. Since he made no mention of cost sharing, it seemed like a simple invitation to come join him. This sounded like such a good opportunity that I accepted his offer, packed a few things and moved to Alexandria. He was right about the apartment but, after I moved in, I discovered that he was living with his girlfriend, who didn't seem to know that this wasn't just a visit. I immediately started checking the want ads to find employment. I wasn't able to stay long before Johan and I had an argument and I was tossed out.

I moved to a motel, but wasn't there more than a few days, before Johan was also asked by the girl friend to leave. He rented an apartment nearby at a nearby apartment complex and invited me to join him. This was still without mention of cost sharing, and I moved in. I hadn't obtained a job, but had been to several promising job interviews. While Johan was out, a Sheriff came to the door. He said I had three days to get one month's rent and the deposit together. Johan's check for the rent had bounced, and they were ready to throw us out of the apartment. I confronted

Johan about the check. He knew he did not have enough money in his checking account and still wrote a bad check. Suddenly, if I wanted to live there, rent had become my responsibility.

This was a great shock because I didn't expect Johan to treat me that way although he had done some sneaky things. Much of my life had been lived on military posts where there was no rent and my parents had not discussed rent with us children. I called Mom for advice and she said she would contact her father to see if he would be able to help me. Grandpa sent me enough money to take care of the deposit and several additional months. I also expected that my retirement money would come to me and help me with my initial expenses. It never came, and I didn't find out until later that Dad, without bothering to say anything to me, had forged my name to the check.

I didn't realize how expensive it was to live in the Washington area. The efficiency apartment cost $475.00 per month including all utilities. This seemed alright until I started finding out about other expenses. In my parent's home I didn't have to worry about the cost of household items, which Mom had paid or about laundry, which Mom had done. Now these costs would be my responsibility if Johan was not going to pay toward the upkeep. Johan's drinking and craziness got to me and he was not contributing. This caused a fierce argument between us and I moved out to a motel in Springfield, Virginia.

I soon found a job as a waitress at a nearby motel's restaurant in Springfield. A short time after I started there, we had a tremendous snow storm. The storm was so bad that it was dangerous to walk and the restaurant invited us to remain at the motel for the night rather than go home in such bad conditions. I tried to start home anyway, but fell and skinned my knee in the parking lot. So I accepted the invitation and bunked in with three other waitresses. We had a merry old time most of the night watching television, talking and playing cards. We were tired the next day but managed to make it through the day alright, possibly because there were few customers with all the snow. However, this work didn't last long because a day or so later I tripped and spilled a coca cola all over a customer. The manager said that I was too clumsy for waitress work and suggested that I try registering with some temporary employment agencies.

I followed his suggestion and managed to keep just busy enough to barely pay the bills. It felt good being on my own. I was just squeaking by and had to scrimp on my medicine in order to make it. Mom phoned from time to time to see how I was doing and started to see through my happy talk. She asked if I was eating right, taking my medicine correctly and seeing doctors. Mom knew how hard things could be, but I never wanted to ask her for additional help, if able to take care of myself. I wanted her to be proud of me. She may have told Dad that I needed help, because Dad phoned to tell me of a friend, who would let me stay in her home. Johan had been evicted from the apartment that I had lived in with him, and Dad had arranged for him to live with this friend. But he had messed up there also, and been tossed out again. It was only because Dad assured her I would be different, that she was willing to have me in her home. I lived there about eight months, and we became very friendly. She even went out of her way to help when I became ill for a few days.

In the midst of working for temporary employment firms, I applied for work at an agency in Washington, D.C. After a few weeks they interviewed and hired me as a clerk. This seemed that it would cover my financial needs and would be the permanent employment I had been looking for. I was hired as a clerk typist and found the people friendly. A coworker named Pam seemed particularly pleasant, and I often ate lunch with her. However, I found my supervisor to be impossible and went back to temp work after about six months.

I soon got a job with a real estate office in northern Virginia supporting over sixty part and full-time agents. Ellen, a million dollar seller, was our best agent and an inspiration to many in real estate sales. As easily the best sales agent in our office she pressed for and received a lot of office support. We became firm friends. I helped her distribute her sales circulars on my own and once on company time. Circular distribution about their own accounts was the responsibility of the individual agents. So the office manager told me not to do that on company time without his permission.

I was the only office member invited to her marriage reception to a very prominent man. I went, even though I feel uncomfortable in crowds. This was more difficult because I'm a short and felt especially conspicuous in the large group of six foot guests who were drinking alcoholic beverages which I can't do because of possible interactions with my medicines. I hadn't expected to feel so frightened and alone and left soon after Ellen greeted me. In the office she asked what had happened to me and was not too happy with my explanation but didn't let it interfere with our friendship.

This lasted for about a year until the start of a new job at a land title company in D.C. as secretary to the settlement attorney. I prepared deeds, titles, contracts, and pushed the examiners to get the paperwork to my boss for processing. This one was especially enjoyable; my supervisor and the other employees were easy to get along with. I even had pleasant phone conversations with my supervisor's wife. It felt as though I had found a home. However, it was destined to last only a little over six months. I resigned because Mom's health had deteriorated badly and the doctors recommended that she move west. They said if she moved to the dryness of Arizona it would help her health. Mom wanted to move to California to be nearer Phil and his family. The doctors said San Diego might do for a short time but Arizona was essential for the long haul.

MCLEAN, VIRGINIA

Mom smoked cigarettes for many years until the damage they cause finally caught up with her. The emphysema was so advanced that she was attached to oxygen most of the time. Unable to work, she was totally dependent on Dad for support. He got a job in northern Virginia in an engineering firm, and my parents moved to McLean to be near Dad's job. After they were there about a year, Mom began to notice that Dad's behavior was changing. She suspected that he was seeing another woman. Mom was too clever for Dad to be able to keep hidden something that important. While he slept, she carefully rummaged through his things, to see what she could find. All of the drawers and closet spaces were clear of suspicious items, but she found some writing paper torn up in small bits in a vase. Mom gathered all the pieces together, assembled them like a picture puzzle, and taped them together.

Mom was so angry and disappointed in my Dad, that she woke him at two a.m. screaming, "What is going on?" They had an awful argument, and Mom phoned me the next morning, crying that Dad was leaving her for someone else. My unbelieving response was, "Don't be crazy he loves you and would never do anything to hurt you. I'll be there to check things out." She had the proof with the letter, and knew him well enough to know what to expect. Within the next few days, I carefully examined my parent's car, and found another letter Dad had written. This one said that his leaving Mom was OK with me, which was an outright lie. Now my parents slept in separate bedrooms.

After a few days, Dad left. He cleaned out the bank account and left her; sick, without food, money or even a telephone in the apartment. He just got up and left! Never said a word to anyone, gone! I remember being so angry with him, that I contacted my friend Ellen, from the real estate company in Virginia, for help in obtaining a lawyer. She said she had a friend, an excellent lawyer, who would get legal support from Dad for Mom. This calmed me since she was very successful in real estate, and had good connections in the legal profession. I moved in with Mom, in order to be as much help as possible, but in a few days it became obvious that this wouldn't be enough. She needed more care than, while working, I could provide. Her doctors told us the climate of the East Coast was too moist for her condition. She would be better off in the dry climate of Arizona. Mom said that she would prefer San Diego to Phoenix. The doctors said San Diego might be alright for a short time, but Phoenix would be much better in the long run. I asked my brothers, Johan and Mike to help support me with Mom's care on such a trip. They were in their early twenties and had not yet established themselves. Barely able to support themselves, they refused. I told them that, if we went to the west coast, this was probably the last time they would see Mom alive. Phil had married recently and was living in Los Angeles, California. He had problems of his own in establishing a new family. Taking care of Mom, in probably the final few years of her life, would be a privilege, but it looked like the pleasure would be all mine.

The lawyer that Ellen contacted was very competent. He obtained judgments in Mom's favor for support. When Dad refused to comply with them, by changing jobs without notifying the court, our lawyer had his private detective find his new employers. Then he went back to court to have Dad's wages garnisheed again. (A garnishment is a court order for the employer of a noncompliant debtor to pay a certain amount out of his wages to the creditor). Each time Dad changed jobs without notifying the court, our lawyer hunted him down. He found Dad's new employer and garnisheed his wages again with extra charges for his effort. This cannot have been helpful in maintaining Dad's continuing desire to look good, and must have put economic strains on his new love life. He must have been even angrier at us, for having him pursued and needing to pay the extra costs, of chasing him along with new court charges.

TO SAN DIEGO, CALIFORNIA

Mom and I decided to move to San Diego. I asked my brothers Johan and Mike again for help but they didn't see how they could be useful and declined. I resigned my job at the title company, cleaned out and closed my bank account. Then, Mom and I flew to San Diego. Pam, who had worked with me at the agency in D.C. and I had become friends. She asked her sister, Kit, who lived in San Diego, to meet us at the airport. Kit helped us find an unfurnished efficiency apartment, which we rented and I started to look for work. We were hungry, and she joined us in a snack of peanut butter and crackers as we sat on the floor. We were almost broke and I asked Kit for some financial help. She said that, as a military wife with limited resources, the best she could do was to order a phone for us in her name until we could afford to pay for one. I scrounged up two light aluminum lounge chairs to sleep on. They were from the apartment complex's swimming pool. I climbed over the tall locked swimming pool fence at night and tossed them back over. The lounge chairs, along with pillows and blankets that we had brought with us, made adequate beds.

Trying to find work in San Diego was very difficult. You had to know someone in order to get a decent even temp jobs, if you could get them, paid poorly. I can't remember finding work there. My savings were rapidly running out and we hadn't started to receive Mom's garnishment support checks from Dad's employers. Money was so short that we had a continuous diet of peanut butter. I called Mom's father for help and he sent us $15,000.00 as a onetime gift to help us through our difficulties. We were in tall cotton! I went to the grocery and bought over two hundred dollars worth of food and other needed consumables. It felt good to pay Kit for the phone costs and have the phone switched to my name. I kept looking unsuccessfully for work.

Within a month Mom's support checks started to arrive and we deposited them into a bank account in Mom's name. We seemed to be better off, although having to dip into the $15,000.00 because the support checks weren't enough to cover expenses. I continued looking for work. Then several checks drawn on Mom's new bank account bounced. We wondered if Johan had somehow gotten some of Mom's checks. But we found out after several days that the bank had made a procedural error. They returned the missing money to our account and wrote letters of apology to the people who had received the bounced checks.

Soon, we received a letter from Dad, with a court order that Dad said he had received. This reduced the support he was required to pay Mom each month from $1200.00 to $400.00. It was on plain paper and had typographical errors. We phoned our lawyer, who said that the court order was a fake, and that a court order would be signed and sealed with an official seal. He informed the judge of Dad's attempt to avoid garnishment. Dad was forced to appear in court to show why he should not be held in contempt of court. Then our lawyer contacted Dad's employer to be sure that he obeyed the judge's order for the full amount of the judgment. The employer may have fired Dad or maybe he just skipped. Either way, suddenly, Dad was working there no longer, and the garnishment checks ceased until our lawyer found his new employer. I kept looking for work and, if I found any, it wasn't successful enough to be able to remember. If there was anything it would have been short term temp work and poorly paid. I was increasingly tired of the work situation in San Diego and started looking at where I would be able to find dependable work. These were hard times because Mom was getting worse. She said she was feeling better, but I knew, from her increasing shortness of breath, that time was running out on her.

LOS ANGELES, CALIFORNIA

My brother, Phil, and his wife, were living in Los Angeles. Phil said that work was better there. Mom wanted to move to be near them even though L A's smog was not good for her, with the congestive heart condition and emphysema. But, she wanted to see them, at least for a while, and I needed work to sustain us. After six months in San Diego, we moved to be near Phil's family and for work. L A's smog was hard on us, so we had to move soon. I didn't drive, so cabs were the way of getting around when there was no public transit, which was most of the time. Mom was able to walk with difficulty, and some walking was good for her. Days I wasn't working, with light smog, Mom and I walked for her health and to shop. We lived close to stores and she said, "I'm getting better, and can do without oxygen," and turned it off. Knowing her increasing shortness of breath showed she was worse; her lack of reality bothered me.

She loved Phil and Virginia, so much that her face glowed every time they came to visit. I loved Mom dearly and was deeply conscious of how much of my life I owed to her. It gave me a good feeling, to know that I was able to bring her this happiness toward the end of her life after all the misery that she had to endure with Dad. However, I resented the fact that he had deserted her and that all of this responsibility had fallen on me.

Dad was still trying to avoid any support whatsoever, as he moved to new jobs without notifying anyone. This meant our lawyer hunting him down to serve his new employer with garnishment papers. We were fortunate that our lawyer was very competent and found him every time. Each time he went back to the judge for additional monies to cover the cost of finding Dad. The judge granted additional judgments and Dad was garnisheed even heavier. The money was sent to our lawyer, but Dad was furious with Mom at being caught. Any hatred that he had for Mom increased enormously as the garnishment made him look badly and financially crimped his life style with his new love.

Getting temp work in Los Angeles was easier than in San Diego, where it was necessary to know someone to get work. There was a lot of competition for jobs in this Navy town with a large naval base, and a lot of military wives supplementing family incomes. Also, there were many poorly paid Mexicans coming into the U. S., which especially suppressed local prevailing wages. In Los Angeles, my temp assignments usually were good, with $500.00-$600.00 weeks. This was enough every week to be comfortable, and I usually spent it all. The steady work required extra effort on my part. In order to have steady temping assignments I learned a number of different computer software packages. Different employers used different software packages and getting assignments meant knowing the particular software being used by the prospective employer.

One of the fun times in L.A. was at a hamburger joint for lunch. When I was seated I noticed a popular movie and television actress at an adjoining table. I asked the waitress about the actress and she confirmed it. I introduced myself, saying that I enjoyed her show. She invited me to eat with her and we chatted for a while. I found her to be a most pleasant person. It made my day.

The smog was bothering Mom and her health was deteriorating. It was time to move to Arizona. So, we collected our things and caught a bus to Phoenix.

MESA, ARIZONA

The trip to Phoenix was not a piece of cake. With Mom sick, we had to have the oxygen machine and bottle on the next seat at the cost of another fare. Mom was still heavily addicted to cigarettes and wanted to smoke when I hooked up the oxygen bottle. This was not allowed by the bus driver, who was afraid of the extra potential for fire with the oxygen and lit cigarette. At one of the bus stations we had almost run out of oxygen. I explained to the manager that Mom needed the oxygen to live, and asked him to allow us to plug our oxygen machine into an electrical outlet. He said no that this would require him to unplug a video game machine. So, I replied, "Fine don't worry about it" and was so angry that I unplugged two or three machines, then plugged in our machine to recharge the bottle. The game machines would all have to be re-programmed the next business day. When he blustered about calling the police I told him that, if lack of oxygen had cost Mom's life, he would have had a lawsuit on his hands, and the popular bus company would have loved the publicity.

We arrived in Phoenix with little of Granddad's money left and had to be very careful with our spending. We spent our first night in a fleabag motel which seemed to do a lot of business with prostitutes. The next day I looked in the papers for an apartment.

There was an ad for an unfurnished apartment on Gilbert Street in the suburb of Mesa. It cost only one hundred dollars to move in and included all utilities, washer & dryer, nice balcony, 2 bedrooms, 2 bathrooms, kitchen and living room We considered this a huge bargain and moved immediately. Since we had no furniture, I climbed the swimming pool fence and borrowed two light aluminum pool lounges as I had in San Diego. Eventually the property manager found out and came to the door to talk to me about it. When she saw Mom's breathing equipment and that we had no furniture, she said we could borrow them as long as we needed them. She also mentioned that she would have appreciated my asking instead of just taking the lounges. I found a temp job and had hopes of finding more although finding work there was difficult.

Mom was seriously ill and I knew that she could not last much longer. But when I heard that our favorite performer, Neil Diamond would be appearing in concert at the Arizona State University Center on in nearby Tempe, I couldn't resist attending. I purchased a ticket and was happy to be at his concert once again. But I couldn't enjoy it this time, because I was worried about having left Mom alone at the apartment, I went home early.

In May, she was in awfully bad shape and it was clear that her time was getting short. Nevertheless, when the end came, it took me by surprise. I had been sleeping next to her and waking up at every little noise. She went into the toilet to relieve herself and had a heart attack while on the commode. I heard her fall and called her but there was no answer. Jumping up, I rushed to her. She had fallen against the tub, gashing her head and was bleeding heavily. I couldn't get her to wake up or completely stop the bleeding and had to leave her to call the emergency squad. After rushing back to her I managed to stop the bleeding and held her in my arms, trying to help as much as I could. The emergency team still didn't come, so I called again, rushed back and held her some more. I reminded her she had said she wouldn't leave me and begged her to hang on.

She told me she saw the most beautiful white light she had ever seen and had to go to it. I could not see it and was devastated to think that she was dying. Much more recently as I have read the bible and have discussed it with my pastor I have learned that this was the light of Jesus which she could see because she was seeing in the spirit. I find it very comforting to know that she was going to be with him. Just after she stopped breathing, they arrived at the door and resuscitated her. She was breathing as we got to the hospital. However, shortly after she arrived in the emergency room the doctor came to tell me that she was dead.

Mom died at the age of sixty from congestive heart failure. We were only in the apartment for a month. I was heartsick; my best friend who had sacrificed so much in raising me had died and I couldn't prevent it. This was really hard after all the moving and trying to get to the right place. I thought that if taken to Arizona and she had her oxygen everything would be ok. She would live!! Her death broke my heart.

I must have said something like, "Now, I have nothing to live for," in front of one of the nurses. When I started to leave the hospital, a doctor tried to talk me into signing myself into the psych ward until I would be more able to deal with Mom's death. I refused and walked out of the hospital to go back to the apartment. As I was walking along, a police officer stopped me and tried to persuade me to return to the hospital. I refused, but he kept talking to me. Finally, he persuaded me to get into the car, after he said that he would get me help, but not return me to the hospital.

He took me to a local crisis center, and they gave me a sedative to help me sleep. Then I phoned Pam and asked her to tell my brothers what had happened. It seemed unbelievable to tell them that Mom had died. I was all wound up, typing on their typewriter, cleaning, doing anything I could to keep busy, thinking this would take my mind off of my misery. Then they gave me the strongest sedative they had, but I still couldn't sleep. Up over seventy two straight hours, I went to my room, and when they didn't see me, they came looking. They found me where I had passed out, on the floor beside the bed. Afraid that I might waken, they put a pillow under my head, a blanket over me and let me sleep there.

When I woke my brother Phil and Virginia were there with Johan and Mike. They brought me back to the apartment and took turns staying with me because they were concerned about what I might do There were too little funds to bury Mom, so Virginia borrowed four thousand dollars from a home finance company for the burial. Johan, Mike, Phil and I agreed to repay a thousand dollars each. It was several years before my part could be paid.

After the burial, I wanted the few mementoes of Mom to be shared equally among us, but Johan tried to take more than seemed right. I limited what he could have, told him that it was my apartment and ordered him out. Then he left for home. I gave most of the rest of Mom's things to Phil, Virginia and Mike, and they went back to California. With all this I couldn't afford a headstone but at least she had a decent burial. It was over ten years before my husband, Dave, and I were able to purchase a headstone for her, but she has one now.

HOMELESSNESS
AND SHELTERS

After Mom died, I couldn't get my act together. I was all alone, with no friends or personal support closer than California or the east coast. Final arrangements for Mom had taken almost all my money and my intense grief made me unable to concentrate. Deciding to go back to the Washington area but with too little money for the trip, I phoned my friend Ellen, whose lawyer had arranged for Mom's support from Dad. She wired me airfare, and I flew back to Dulles Airport near Washington, D. C. With too little money for rent, and ashamed to approach Ellen for more money, I camped out at Dulles. The first night security guards wanted to know what I was doing there and I told them that I was waiting for a friend. Still later that night, a guard loaned me a blanket and let me sleep in a secluded area under a row of seats. But this could continue for only so long.

After another day or so, I made my way to Rockville, Maryland to see Pam, with whom I had become friends at the D. C. agency. This was to ask her to let me stay with her while I was trying to get on my feet. I arrived at her home in Rockville tired, bedraggled and dirty. It was raining and no one was home. A neighbor saw me, stuck outside in the rain, and had mercy on me. She invited me in, fed me, and allowed me to clean up and wait there until Pam arrived home. When she arrived and consulted with her husband and some friends she decided that a guest in the shape I was in, for an unknown length of time, would not be something they could manage.

Then she took me to a shelter in Rockville, where I stayed for about two months. I was in terrible emotional shape, and unable to gather myself together enough to do a decent interview, let alone work. The shelter wasn't too bad a place under the circumstances. It provided three meals a day and counseling to help me emotionally. While there, one of the other clients had a grand mal seizure. Since the staff didn't know what to do, I took over. I asked them to bring me a pillow for her head and, gently but firmly, held her on the floor, so she wouldn't get hurt by the convulsions. They asked me about helping her breathe and I told them that she'd be able to breathe without assistance. When the convulsions ceased and she came to, I helped her get cleaned up from the involuntary passing of her bowels and got her clothes washed. When they asked how I knew all this, I explained that I had epilepsy. A staff member thanked me for the help. It felt good to be able to do something useful.

About the end of my second month there, I phoned Dad for help to get on my feet. He said fifty dollars, one time only, was the best that he could do and wired the money. When the management saw the check they said that it would have to be put in their account in order for me to stay there. This was to provide security for it, but I was in no condition to trust anyone, and decided that I would try to make other arrangements. When I left they warned me that if I went it would be a year before I could return.

I decided that, if the shelter was going to take my money, at least I could have one good night's sleep before going back to the noise of shelters. I rented a room for one night from a motel, down Rockville Pike toward Washington, D. C. The room had a bath, free television and cost sixty dollars, which was almost all that I had. When I told the manager that I was hungry and nearly out of money, he authorized a complimentary breakfast for the following morning. The next day I caught a bus to Washington to try to find food, shelter and work. Food and shelter were first, because I was in such bad emotional shape that I couldn't hold even a temp job. This forced me to beg on the streets, use homeless shelters for a place to sleep and soup kitchens for most meals.

That day, I found another shelter, where I stayed only one night because of the rats and mice that they had then. Also, I left because I objected to another client wanting to share my bed with me. After that, I went to a Christian shelter, in Washington. It too, had some very friendly clients, and I started carrying a knife for my protection and to discourage client advances. This shelter only provided meals on weekends and then, only breakfast and supper. I soon learned to panhandle (beg). Hunger will teach that.

Before long, I heard of two soup kitchens. Neither was close to where I was living and each was difficult to get to. But in order to eat, I had to be there at mealtime, which was not always possible. So, without work, for money, I still needed to pan handle for food, bus fare and personal items, such as soap and toothpaste, which are important in a job search.

One Sunday on the way to one of the soup kitchens I met a woman going to church who invited me to come with her. I accepted and we went. Soon afterward she invited me to lunch at her home where she asked if I wanted to freshen up. I said yes and she allowed me to take a bath in the Jacuzzi in the master bath room. Then she told me that if I needed to rest it was OK and she would wake me when lunch was ready. I was very tired and slept for a while in the huge bed in the master bed room. Since the shelter did not serve food I gratefully accepted her wonderful meal. She seemed to be happy to provide these free services and said that it was normal for her and her husband to help homeless people in what seemed to me to be a beautiful home. After I got out of homelessness, perhaps six months, I went back to what I thought was the house but couldn't find it. A person, who I thought was a neighbor, said that the woman had moved and the house was not what I remembered but had been a rundown dump for many years. I wondered if we were we talking about the same person and place remembering it as lovely a home as I had seen. I had come to bring some money for the kindness shown me but she was gone and I had no idea where. This felt a little like the poem, "Footprints" where there was only set of "footprints" in the sand and it was Jesus' because he carried a person through a rough time. This time I had been the person carried.

The shelters that I knew had similar objectives: to house the homeless safely and help them work their way off the streets. They had somewhat different but similar rules. All of them prohibited drugs, alcohol, and violence. The services that the shelters provided and how they managed those services varied. The levels of competence also varied between and within shelters. They insisted that adults be out looking for work or working by a certain time each work day, and that children be in school, when school was in session. But not all of them were equipped to house children. When they were able to provide counseling or training, attending these activities was acceptable instead of work or looking for work. They insisted that clients produce evidence of performance, and not return to the shelter, until a specified time daily. Also they had rules about what time clients had to return, in order to be housed at night, although they allowed exceptions based on formal arrangements related to work.

These shelters struggled on limited budgets, to provide as many beds as possible, to as many clients as they could handle, and to provide as many services as they could, to help clients escape from homelessness. Because of this their staffs were frequently spread thinly in old buildings. They had to depend on other shelters, related organizations and volunteers to provide support services which they couldn't afford. They did the best that they could to perform their missions with their limited resources. With these limitations, their ability to deliver quality service was sometimes limited. I believe that it was largely because of this that sometimes pest control was poor and other services were of uneven quality. It was noisy at night in every shelter, which was a natural result of housing such troubled clients. Also, with low wages, the abilities and skills of employees and volunteers were sometimes limited. They did their best to provide a safe place to help troubled people but under these circumstances it was difficult and I didn't feel safe in the shelters.

I tried to get temp work, while in the shelters but, distraught with grief for the first few weeks, was unable to concentrate well enough, to hold the few jobs, for which I was able to qualify. At first, going through interviews, without crying, was more than I could handle. However, with time and counseling from shelter staff and organizations that they referred me to, I gradually began to regain my composure and ability to concentrate. Most of my shelter experience was at a shelter run by a Christian organization. It wasn't until I was there for a while, that I was able to get and hold a job. Gradually, I started back with the temp services again, earning money, instead of pan handling for the little needed for bus fare to the soup kitchens, interviews, etc.

With an income came money problems. Mom had taught me to be compassionate and generous. The feelings of unworthiness that troubled me from childhood were magnified with homelessness, and I considered others better than myself. These feelings made me particularly vulnerable to being scammed by other homeless people used to living by their wits. When other shelter mates told me their hard luck stories I gave or loaned them money that I never saw again. Also, I was naïve and fell for more involved scams. One shelter mate woke me in the middle of the night, with a story that she had seen another in my locker, and suggested putting my things in her locker, for safekeeping. I did, and the next morning my stuff was there, but my money was gone and the shelter mate, too. These incidents sometimes left me without money for food or bus fare and I had to pan handle again to be able to eat. When the shelter manager noticed that I seemed hungry, though working, she wanted to know why. I told her about giving my money away but refused to tell to whom I had given it, lest they be expelled.

As a result of these experiences, I arranged with Pam, who was still working nearby at the D C agency to hold my money and just give me a minimum to take care of immediate needs. This seemed to work alright, but was not foolproof. One time, Pam had just given me ten dollars of my money. When I left the building where Pam worked, a homeless acquaintance asked me for a dollar. Since I had only the ten dollar bill, she said that she would take it and bring me the change. She accepted the ten and disappeared. Then I went back to Pam again. She was angry that I had been so foolish, and told me not to do that again. I learned my lesson and didn't let people take my money to bring me change any more. This was not the only time that Pam was unhappy with me. Occasionally, when I went to see her, other street people would follow me into the offices. They sometimes were poorly clothed and/or had bare feet, which wasn't the ideal style for a business office. Since they had come more or less with me, office people associated me with this work distraction. So I learned to be more careful, entering offices and to be sure to present as good an appearance as possible.

Beside housing me the Christian shelter was giving me counseling, but, after I tried to commit suicide by cutting my wrist with a knife a couple of times, they decided that I needed help from people more specialized in working with that kind of problem. They talked with me about this and referred me to a Crisis Center which had a few rooms for clients in need of their specialized services. I was there for several weeks. While I had come to appreciate the manager at the shelter, I liked the change at the Crisis Center. This was partly because they provided meals, and on days when the cook was off, gave vouchers for meals at a nearby restaurant. While there I met a woman, whom I'll call Jane, who started taking me to a weekly home Bible study that she had just found in a nearby town. I discovered that I was starting to understand the Bible more, and really enjoyed the healing messages in it. Also, I liked the emotional and spiritual support, and the chance to socialize with people who asked nothing of me, other than to be, the best me that I could be. After a while, I was working pretty regularly and had saved enough money with Pam, to try and find private housing. So, I started looking in the local papers at ads placed by people in apartments who were looking for roommates.

THE POST SHELTER APARTMENT

The Washington Post had an advertisement placed by a woman named Sally who lived in an apartment in Silver Spring, Maryland. I phoned and met with her that night and paid two month's rent on the room. Since my shelter friend Jane had no place to live, I asked Sally if it would be alright for Jane to come live with us as my guest. Sally said that it would be alright and Jane moved into Sally's apartment along with me. This was without paying anything because she wasn't working. Shortly, her son from farther north in Maryland came to visit. He was out of work and stayed on. We kept going to the weekly Bible study and Sally sometimes joined us.

Within a few weeks, another son, his wife, their son and dog came from Virginia to live with us. The apartment was now heavily overcrowded. My room was occupied by Jane, her son from Virginia, with his wife, son and dog, and I was sleeping on the floor in the living room. The couch in the living room was occupied by her other son. Sally said that, because of the crowd, bathroom time was limited to fifteen minutes. The food bill was enormous; as was the phone bill and they were paying nothing. I was paying it all. I asked Jane if they could spare $100.00 a month for rent. She told me that I was being unreasonable and there'd be no way. I'd made a mess of things and didn't know how to fix it. When asked to leave, they said no and that I couldn't make them do it. I never thought of contacting the police to remove them. Desperate, I went to my room, closed the door, pushed the chest against it as a barricade and sat there a little while, thinking about what to do. They started pounding on the door and trying to push it open. I had jumped out of windows at home, when I was younger, and decided to do it now, to get away from this mess. However, there was another problem; this was the third floor.

I pushed out the screen and jumped. After landing on the ground I couldn't get up. I could move my legs, but not stand. I tried, but had lots of pain. Lying there, I could hear scrambling around in my room and saw them come to the window. When they looked out, there was more commotion. In a few minutes a police officer asked me if I could move and if I had tried to commit suicide. I moved my legs and told him that I couldn't stand up and that suicide had never entered my mind. He called the emergency squad and they hauled me to a local hospital.

HOSPITALIZATION

At the hospital, as the initial shock wore off, the pain in my back became unbearable. I was sedated with Morphine, x-rayed and given an M R I to reveal the further extent of my injuries. The x-ray and M R I displayed a broken lower back with severe trauma throughout the area. After arriving at my room they placed me in traction and, within the first few days, ordered a plastic body cast. It extended from just below my shoulders to below my crushed tail bone. At first I had to lie flat on my back, but after a few weeks was permitted to sit up. I was knocked out for the first day or so and remained groggy from the morphine for a longer period of time. At first, I was extremely thirsty, allowed only a few sips of water to drink, and fed intravenously. A hospital admissions clerk soon came, and helped file for medical assistance and Supplementary Social Security Income because of my injury.

I soon started receiving visitors from the Bible study, especially Ann, the lady in whose home the Bible study was held, and Dave, the Bible study leader. I remember Pam, from the D C agency, visiting. She was angry that I was foolish enough to jump from a third floor window. Ann and Dave visited several times. They brought me ice water and Dave brought me an entire pitcher, because I couldn't seem to get enough. I was in the local hospital almost six weeks, when I heard that the State of Maryland was paying my hospital costs of about twenty five thousand dollars for my stay there. They wanted to transfer me to a state hospital as soon as possible in order to lower costs.

Probably because of my jumping out of the third floor window, they chose a mental hospital, in Maryland. I didn't like that idea and phoned for Dave to visit, thinking that he might let me stay at his home, since he lived alone and had two extra bedrooms. When he arrived I asked him about this but he said he wasn't equipped to help me in my physical condition. I tried to get up to show him I could walk, but had been in bed so long, that my muscles had shrunk and I was having a difficult time getting off the bed. (Dave told me later that I moved like a crab trying to skitter off the bed). While I was trying to get up he walked down the hall and left the building. I kept screaming for him because of no desire to go to the mental hospital. I can't have been thinking clearly because I staggered to a stair door in a string tie hospital gown trying to escape before a nurse asked what I was doing. I said, going to get ice water and slowly wobbled back to my room.

When I arrived at the mental hospital I found an entirely different atmosphere. In the local hospital, I had been in a room with two beds in the part of the hospital devoted to severe body injuries. Now everything was more severely regimented, and doors were locked, so that I couldn't get out of that section of the hospital, even if I were mobile. Not only that; they had very limited visiting hours, and visitors had to ring at the front door to be escorted. From there they were taken to another locked door into my section. I had a private room that opened into a day room used by perhaps thirty other patients. All were being treated for their particular emotional and/or psychiatric problems. The patients varied from seeming normal to somewhat weird, but had one thing in common; all were somewhat subdued. I assume that the staff administered calming sedatives to keep everyone, peaceful and easier to control. Obviously, medications were closely guarded and administered on schedules established by the doctors. As soon as I arrived the doctors added another sedating medication to my regimen. I don't remember what it was, but it probably was the one keeping all the other patients calm. It was very strong and affected my vision. I was unable to complete their questionnaire, from inability to read the print.

I was angry with Dave, and refused to see him when he came to visit the day after my arrival, because I felt that, if he had rented me a room, I would not have been in a mental hospital. However, after a few days, he returned, and with me cooled off, we had a pleasant visit. He helped me complete the questionnaire that I still couldn't read because of the effect of the new sedative. He told me that, when I was discharged and more able to get around, if I was unable to find another place, he would allow me to stay at his home for one month.

I hated the confinement and was still angry at being there. Furthermore, the heavy sedative, which interfered with my vision, made me furious. But the doctors insisted on dosing me with it. I refused to take it, or to attend required group meetings until they took me off the sedative. They responded by putting me in restraints tied to the bed and fed it to me intravenously. This was a fine kettle of fish. Now, what to do? I thought about it, and noticed that the toilet in my room locked on the inside, but had no way to be opened from the bedroom side. I told the nurse that I had to go to the toilet, and she let me out of my restraints. Once in the toilet, I locked the door and wouldn't come out. When nurses ordered me to come out, I refused until it was agreed that I be taken off restraints, and the sedative which was limiting my vision. I pointed out that I had plenty of water, toilet paper and a place to relieve myself. I could last for a long time, although without my seizure medicine, it might get a little rough. Finally a doctor promised to remove the restraints and stop the offending sedative. I didn't trust them and still wouldn't unlock the door. This situation continued for several hours until my doctor came, and assured me that I wouldn't have to take the sedative or be in restraints. In return, I agreed to attend the group meetings, and the confrontation was over. They transferred me to a semiprivate room with a different toilet arrangement.

By this time, having been in bed or in a wheel chair for so long enough left me unable to walk. My doctor said, "You'll never be able to walk." I said, "I will," and started trying to do it despite being in the full body cast. This started by leaning on the table in my room for support. While trying to walk around it, I fell and had a hard time getting up. The doctor wouldn't let the nurses help me, and insisted that I get up by myself. It wasn't easy but I managed it and kept trying to walk. Then the nurses, helped get me out of the wheel chair to practice with a four legged walker. It wasn't fun using it, but helped me progress to walking with a cane. Finally, I graduated to unassisted walking, although somewhat stiffly at first.

LAYTONIA DRIVE

The day came when the doctors at the mental hospital were ready to release me, and I called Dave to come get me. I hadn't made any real efforts to find other places to live because the only choices, without money for food or rent, seemed to be the shelters, and I had already had my fill of them. So, I told Dave that I couldn't find anything else, and he came to pick me up. Dave's home near Rockville was a three bedroom, one and a half bath townhouse and I had my own room. He didn't drink coffee and wouldn't buy me any which really annoyed me, but I had to go without it because I had no money. After all, he was supplying both food and shelter for free, so I pretty much kept quiet about the coffee. I had no money for transportation, was in the plastic body cast from shoulders to tailbone and had difficulty walking. It was impossible to get out of Dave's home within the original month he had said that I could stay there. So he extended the time for me to leave.

He attended church regularly and insisted on my going with him at least once. We argued about it, but he said without my going at least once, I couldn't live there. I tried it, liked the music, worship, and teaching and continued attending.

The move to Dave's was not all sweetness and light. Upon arrival, I was angry about things in general and we had some very severe arguments. One time he slapped me in order to shock me out of an extremely bad argument, but that only made me angrier and he said that he'd never do it again. He has been good to his word although I tried to goad him into slapping again to test him. In the middle of another argument, he tried to get to the phone to have people from Sykesville come get me. I managed to disconnect the telephone jack and we both calmed down enough to come to some agreements.

As time passed and we got used to one another's ways, things smoothed out considerably. I was enjoying the neighborhood animals; my back was getting stronger, and hurting less. Visits to the county subsidized clinic were decreasing and counseling was at a state subsidized rate. As my back improved I took public transportation to medical appointments, light shopping and job interviews, scheduled by phone. Dave took me to these activities, when they didn't interfere with his work. After a while, it was alright to remove the cast at night, but still essential to wear it while I was on my feet, or exerting myself in any way. As you may imagine it was most uncomfortable in the summer heat, when it was hot, chafed and itched. Scratching was impossible in most locations because of the hard plastic. You might know, just as the cooler temperatures of fall made the cast less uncomfortable I was able to stop wearing it entirely.

After living at Dave's a few weeks, my Social Security Disability checks started coming and I was able to buy a coffee maker, coffee and filters, which felt a lot better. What a relief! At that time living with him and going through caffeine withdrawal seemed more than I could stand. Also, unbeknown to Dave, I started buying pet food for the cute little barrel of a Norwich terrier named Killer that lived next door. An animal lover, I couldn't resist feeding him and other animals in the neighborhood. I had to keep this a secret because Dave's purpose for letting me live there was to help me get reestablished and out on my own. He didn't discover my animal feeding until I told him about it much later although he mentioned that animals seemed to be hanging around the yard. I suggested my paying rent out of the Social Security Dependency money. He said to save it to build enough of a nest egg to get my own place as soon as I could find work. Later, he said rent refusal also was so that it would be easier to get rid of me if I got too comfortable with the arrangement and didn't make reasonable efforts to get work. I didn't like the idea of living on charity if I could avoid it, so I snuck a few of his bank deposit slips and put money in his bank account. Since I had put money in his account, he wouldn't be able to prove that I wasn't paying rent. Anything, to buy time! He was careless with his account and never noticed.

Some of my shelter friends, who had lived with me at the apartment, were delaying returning my television set and some other miscellaneous things from a nearby state where they had moved after they were tossed out. Dave and I went on a Saturday and retrieved them. With my SSI support coming in monthly, I had enough money to have other belongings shipped from Phil's home on the west coast. Having all of my things was like having an early Christmas in November.

I had not been allowed to go swimming alone and doctors had instructed my parents that someone always needed to be with me while swimming. As a result I was afraid of the water. But, hearing Dave and his grandchildren talk about their good times swimming, spurred my interest. So when they invited me to go with them to a lake in a state park, I accepted and bought a bathing suit. They explained that, with my plumpness, I would certainly float well, and that they would be with me all the time in the water. Dave alerted the lifeguard that I had epilepsy, although without a seizure in several years. I was fearful at first, but after a short time in the water and finding my buoyancy to be true, I enjoyed it. On the way home I thought about how gracious God had been to me over the years in the midst of all my problems.

One day my friend, Ann, and I went shopping to the local K-Mart store. While there, she received a cell phone call and started rushing me along. I asked her what was wrong and she said she had a party to go to. I asked if I could go, but she said, "Not this time." She continued rushing me, and I asked her the time of the party. She said it was later in the evening. I didn't understand why she was in such a hurry. Dave had called her cell phone to tell her that my brother, Mike had committed suicide and to bring me home immediately because Dad was there waiting to tell me about it. When I saw Dad, I asked him if he was ok and he told me "Yes." Then I asked him what was wrong, and he told me of Mike's death. Dad had tried to help Mike who sometimes had suffered from severe depression, but had been unsuccessful. Mike died at the age of twenty eight. I realize a person is not supposed to have family favorites, but Mike was my favorite brother. He had a wonderful personality and a loving way about him (after he got his tongue clipped, something else before). Mike could play the piano, even simple classical pieces, without reading a note and loved to oil paint. He could go into a room, remember how it looked, and paint it accurately when we got home. He was just amazing! I always felt that he was strong, and that anything I told him in confidence would be kept secret. Perhaps he couldn't afford to buy the medicine that he took for depression. His suicide devastated me and I still miss him.

ATLANTIC CITY TRIP, SUMMER

Dave had been telling me about a wonderful sub sandwich shop in Atlantic City, and I wanted to see the casinos. It would be fun to take the ferry from Lewes, Delaware to Cape May, New Jersey, and to make the sub shop and a casino part of a Saturday trip. We rose early and drove east past Annapolis, on the Chesapeake Bay Bridge, to the eastern shore of Maryland. Continuing across Maryland to Lewes, Delaware, we ferried the mouth of Delaware Bay to Cape May and we fed the sea gulls with bits of bread. There were clouds of them, competing to catch the bits in the air. Watching their acrobatic flying was fun. With exhausted bread we went into the onboard restaurant and Dave suggested brunch. Without the distraction of the gulls, I noticed that the water was a little rough with the large ferry rolling slightly from side to side. This made me feel uncomfortable and I refused fried shrimp, but had a cola to settle my stomach.

While eating we met two older women, traveling to the Atlantic City casinos. They said they took this gambling trip often. One said she enjoyed the excitement of gambling, and came as often as she could. She revealed that gambling had alienated her from her husband and children, and that she had lost her home. Later, Dave said he hates gambling. He doesn't want to lose his own money, disapproves of enterprises which take advantage of people's addictions, and doesn't want their money. Nevertheless he agreed to introduce me to one of the casinos in Atlantic City.

First, we walked along the Cape May beach, enjoying the scenery and looking for sea shells. He told me to watch out for the waves because, if fooled, you can get soaked. Walking along the water's edge, waves chased us. There were areas with large boulders, and while I was making my way through some of these large rocks one of the waves approached. I thought rocks would protect me. Wow! Was I wrong! The wave splashed through the rocks and I was soaked all the up to my waist. Dave took me to a small store on the board walk to buy a change of clothes. They didn't have a fitting room, so I had to change in the car under a large beach towel. Dave seemed to think the whole thing was funny and jokingly called me a hussy.

We drove to Atlantic City, where he took me to a casino. Because Dave was trying to help me get on my economic feet, we agreed to limit my gambling money to one dollar. When I told an employee that this was a new thing for me, and asked him how to operate a slot machine he took me to a vacant machine and showed me. I put my quarters in and got back a dollar and a half. Dave said that this could have been a set up to get me thinking that winning money would be this easy. So we stuck with the plan to only gamble one dollar and left.

We went to a sub shop on Arctic Avenue. The subs were new to me. The rolls were narrow, crunchy and baked fresh every hour at a Sicilian bakery around the corner. They hollowed them out, before filling them with choices, of a variety of foreign and domestic sliced cheeses and meats. Lettuce, tomato and many other tasty vegetables and sauces were available to go with the meats and cheeses. They had a huge variety of sandwiches but we were satisfied with the Italian cold cut subs. Then we headed home vie the Delaware Memorial bridge and Interstate.95.

This time was not all sweetness and light. Looking for work was tough and discouraging. Nothing seemed available until a newspaper ad for a job fair.

A LOCAL UNIVERSITY

A recruiter of a local university invited me to interview at their campus the day after the job fair. It was cold, in December, and I wore jeans under my skirt to keep my legs warm at the bus stops planning to take the jeans off before the interview. Unexpectedly I met the interviewer in the hall before getting a chance to make the change. She didn't seem to be bothered about the jeans, and allowed me to go to the toilet and remove them, as planned. She said that she would be my supervisor and, to my amazement, hired me. It was a great day; I was back working fulltime.

She described the office and its functions before directing me to someone else for introductions to the staff. They were very friendly and made me feel comfortable. As time went by I became proficient at my job, and learned to accommodate the moods of my supervisor. Her good and bad days seemed to reflect what was happening in her home life. I had difficulty accepting the heavy physical work that she performed. However, she gradually persuaded me that, in this particular organization, she was expected to carry her part of the load. She said her grades would be poor if she kept begging for help all the time. Overall she was a good supervisor although her moodiness got to me at times. I made firm friends there, including the person who had shown me around. She turned out to be a new, born again Christian and we had interesting discussions during our lunch hours about our religious points of view. She believed that interest in popular music was sinful, and that Christians should listen strictly to religious music. I wasn't ready for that, but, continuation of my religious journey has generally produced more satisfaction with religious than popular music. She never persuaded me that all secular music is sinful, and I still listen to popular music without feeling guilty.

After a while, some of my supervisor's moods and unfair comments started to get under my skin. I was blessed that about that time an experienced educator joined our section. He was a psychiatrist and deeply committed Christian. We usually arrived before time to start work to discuss our views on human relationships in light of our shared beliefs. He helped me work through my resentments about the things which I considered unfair about my supervisor's directions and comments. After a while I had the opportunity to help him strengthen his computer skills and did some library research for him in addition to my regular assigned duties. We became very good friends and I gradually told him much of my history including the epilepsy and homelessness.

Later, I returned from a three day weekend to an empty office, because they were away on field practice for the week and discovered an open envelope on my supervisor's desk. It contained a large sum of cash for expenses at the field practice. It was the most money I had ever found, and, in my mind, I had it spent. You know that old saying, 'finders keepers, losers weepers.' I had spoken to her about the danger of leaving cash in plain view, but she had a lot on her mind in preparing for the practice and forgot. I locked the money in my desk drawer, but a day or so later one of the secretaries decided to make a copy of my desk key. With the security risk that this presented I decided to report the forgotten cash immediately rather than wait for their return. Keeping the information at the lowest level in order to avoid as much difficulty as possible for my supervisor seemed the way to go. I went to a supervisor lower in responsibility than my supervisor's and asked to speak with her privately. She said of course; closing the door and the blinds to her office, I dumped all the money on her desk and mentioned finding the money. She couldn't believe it and wanted to know where the money came from. I told her and of warning my supervisor about leaving cash out, but not continuing to press it because of not wanting to irritate her. Then I obtained this supervisor's signature on a receipt, with a statement of the amount and where it was found. This never produced a word about it, or any indication of appreciation. Possibly this supervisor claimed to have discovered the money in order to avoid possible embarrassment for my boss for having her subordinate discover her mistake. Sometime after this she received a promotion, so I guess that it wasn't held against her.

My friend, the psychiatrist, was teaching the students about the need for respect and consideration for the people they served, and also the need to be careful with their own finances. He believed that book learning didn't have the impact of face to face contact with people who had experienced life's difficulties. Because of this he asked me to participate in a program on homelessness by describing my experiences and answering questions afterward. The idea of public speaking didn't seem like much fun, even less about a past of which I was not too fond, in front of a class of university students. However, he persuaded me that it would be helpful. Although frightening at first, it went pretty well. Some of them told me that they were going to start savings accounts as the result of my talk, which was satisfying.

Later, my supervisor transferred and a new person replaced her. She had never asked me to do anything improper, but I felt her replacement did. When he asked me to backdate my performance evaluation, I told him that I wouldn't do it, that the evaluation should have been presented to me in a timely manner. If, early on, he asked me to do something inappropriate to escape looking inefficient, I could only imagine what life would be like continuing to work for him. After this disagreement I started looking for another job.

During this time major changes were taking place in my family's life. Phil and Virginia had been married in Pomona, California and had a daughter, whom Phil wanted to name Laura Terri. I felt highly complemented but suggested the substitution of Danielle for Terri in honor of our dead baby sister. The marriage didn't last. Phil and his wife were divorced, because Virginia was the only one working and Phil, addicted at that time to recreational drugs, was at home to look after their new baby. It wasn't working. When Virginia found him passed out rather than caring for a crying Laura the marriage ended. It was sad to know that things had gotten so bad. In time, this resulted in Phil taking a good look at his behavior and deciding to change because he was in no condition to be a proper parent. After a while, Virginia remarried. I had been worried about what was going to happen to them and was happy to know that Virginia and Laura were going to be taken care of.

GRANDPA'S DEATH

Sometime in the summer of 1991 I received a phone call from social services in Charleston, South Carolina that Grandpa wasn't able to take care of himself. They wanted me and to come and either get him, and take care of him. With the amount of work I had on my plate I declined. I told them that if he wanted to move up here and stay in a retirement home that would be fine, but he could not stay with me. Apparently they then contacted my brother, Johan, who, knowing that Grandpa had set up a retirement with a pension from the Navy and savings in some banks, decided that this could be a good thing.

I heard no more about it, until receiving another phone call, this time from the executor of Grandpa's estate. He told me of Grandpa's death, and the need to come arrange his funeral and burial. Johan had left and I was the nearest relative who might be willing to come take care of it. Dave and I drove down and found that there was no money for any of this. Somehow, Grandpa's savings had disappeared. Fortunately, grandpa's Lodge had a fund to contribute toward the burials of members and his fellow members contributed liberally to help with funeral expenses. With their help we were able to have a funeral and have him cremated.

We couldn't afford a casket and regular burial. His Naval career provided a burial plot for his ashes.

This wasn't the end of it. We drove back to clean his apartment and dispose of the items of clothing and furniture that Johan hadn't taken. We met a friend of Johan's who had roomed with him at Grandpa's. He told us that Johan had talked Grandpa into taking out a loan and that all the money was gone. Also that when Johan left, the large new television went with him. The executor of Grandpa's estate told us that Grandpa had willed me the entire twenty thousand dollar estate. Of course that didn't mean much with none of it left. This left me believing that Johan had probably done it to me again.

Dave and I rented a trailer and picked up a few odds and ends such as used clothes and the broken clothes dryer that Dave was able to fix up for our use. They cluttered up the house for a while until we were able to work them into the scheme of things. We still have some of his old handkerchiefs. It feels good to know that Grandpa understood and valued the way I had taken care of his daughter, in her extended terminal illness. That he had tried to leave me everything he owned was proof of his appreciation, even if the money was gone.

NIAGARA FALLS TRIP

Dave often spoke of the majestic beauty of Niagara Falls. He had driven there several times through Friday nights, arriving the next morning, for eight or nine hours of sightseeing. This appealed to me and our small Bible study group. Six of us left in his Toyota minivan about ten p.m. on a Friday night. It was to be a Saturday of sightseeing at the falls with my new Canon thirty five millimeter point and shoot camera. Dave drove with me seated beside him. I was tasked with making sure that he didn't fall asleep. Unfortunately I drifted off around six a, m. on the nearly empty road. Dave was sleepy enough to drive off onto a rough trash laden median strip. The roughness of the ground woke us and we all started yelling at him to wake up and stop the van. He got back on the road and continued driving. This didn't last long, because the median was full of nails which soon flattened two of our tires. Dave changed one, and took the other along the road to a gas station, where he had it repaired and brought it back to continue our trip. While he was getting the tire repaired, Harry went into the nearby woods to relieve himself and returned, well bitten by mosquitoes. With the tire installed, we got back on the road with perhaps the loss of an hour and a half.

There were no more misadventures, and before long we crossed through customs into Canada because the best views of the famous Horse Shoe Falls are from the Canadian side of the river. We started the morning taking pictures and enjoying the natural beauty. The roar of the falls, which could be heard for several miles, was impressive, as was the raw power of the huge volume of water cascading over the rocks before the long drop to the huge pool below. We walked in plastic ponchos provided by a tour, through a tunnel to the lookout under the falls, through the falling water just a few feet in front of us. The tunnel continued to an observation deck beside this section of the falls, where we could view the falling water, up close from the side. Beside the loud roar of the falls, we felt the vibration caused by the tremendous mass of falling water and appreciated the ponchos because of the heavy mist and spray blown by air displaced by the water. I should mention that travel from the USA into Canada today requires passports.

We had a great time. I found a quaint gift shop, which allowed me to buy souvenirs. To this day, I have plastic placemats of Niagara Falls. It would be fun to make that trip again. Scenic travel is a blast! When younger, I tired of the traveling gypsy life of the military. Being in one place and having permanent friends became precious, but I also enjoy scenic travel with Dave. My new digital single lens reflex thirty five millimeter camera made it all the sweeter. It also makes great pictures of local clouds and flowers but I'm eager to get back on the road to capture images with my new and greatly improved equipment.

OUR MARRIAGE

Dave and I were married on September 26, 1992 at our very large nondenominational church. The senior pastor, who had started the church with his wife over twenty years earlier, performed the ceremony with only ten people present: the pastor, an assistant pastor with his wife, the building superintendent, our photographer with his assistant, my bridesmaid (to help with my dress) and her husband, Dave and me. The reason for the small wedding was because Dave knew that his four children, who were all within ten years of my age, knew of my homelessness but didn't know me. He requested we be married without their knowledge because he didn't want them to be giving him advice which might cause problems in our future relationships with them. This meant that they would be hurt if we had my family and others there and severely limited the number of possible invitations. I phoned Dad the day before the wedding to inform him. Despite my explanation, he was upset at the last minute notice and that he wasn't invited.

After several weeks we went on a two week sightseeing/ camping honeymoon into Nova Scotia. Dave had outfitted his empty work van with sofa cushions for beds and curtains for privacy. We had the usual camping supplies of gasoline stove, pots and pans, etc. and plenty of blankets. Before we left Dave mailed a letter to each of his four children informing them of our marriage and honeymoon. It said that we would like to get together to celebrate our marriage after we returned. The first night we pulled into a campground in Vermont that had cabins for rent. It was rustically beautiful and romantic with its own lake. The night was overcast and it started raining after we retired. I was snug in one single bed with Dave in another. Then rain started leaking through the roof right on him. He moved three times before he found a dry area to sleep under. In the morning the rain had stopped, leaving a fresh clean fragrance, and after breakfast we walked around the lake taking pictures. When we left, the campground operator gave us a fifty per cent rain leak discount and told us that we had spent the last possible night at the camp because it was closing that day until next season.

Our next night, we camped in our first Nova Scotia campground. It was drizzling lightly but not enough to spoil our appreciation of the great natural beauty of the autumn leaves that we had been passing through or our sense of adventure and fun. This night was so warm that we didn't need blankets and found it difficult to keep from sweating. But our sense of adventure was undiminished and the heat and light drizzle were only minor irritants. After all this time, the nightly accommodations have run together in our memories, but they varied from renting motel rooms on several nights to camping in the van one night when it got so cold that there was ice on the inside of the windows from the moisture of our breaths. Even that cold, our ample blankets kept us warm, and we enjoyed the contrast with the first night in Nova Scotia when we were perspiring. One additional camp experience stands out in the memories of our honeymoon. Canadians celebrate Thanksgiving as we do in the U. S. A., but on a different date. Our campground hostess made us the present of a delicious homemade pumpkin pie to celebrate their Thanksgiving.

We have many wonderful memories of Nova Scotia. Our first major individual sightseeing goal was the Cabot Trail, roughly two hundred eighty miles of road around Cape Breton Island. We were aiming to particularly enjoy the northernmost forty or fifty miles which go along the edge of Cape Breton Highlands National Park. This part is very hilly and rugged, with the road sometimes down a little above high tide, and other times high up, along a bluff with plenty of ups and downs to match the topography. The country is rough and heavily forested and the visions of the autumnal leaf colors on right side and ocean splashing on the large rocks and small rock strewn beaches on the left have not been forgotten. Also it has small rocky creeks and streams splashing out of the forests in some cases fairly near the road and others way down below. This was particularly visually exciting against the beautiful rich gold, orange and red fall deciduous tree colors combined with evergreens.

Once we left the park the area was still sparsely settled, with occasional little hamlets' enough flat shoreline to encourage vacation housing. This was just past the prime leaf color time, but still gorgeous. We left the park as evening was well advanced and wished that there was both more time and more of it to enjoy. Our timing had been good, as we had limited our time, earlier in the day, to park off the road, enjoy a walk on the rocky beach and play with the smooth rocks shaped by the waves. This allowed us to complete the most rugged and visually interesting part of the trail as darkness fell.

We spent that night at a motel, and the next day visited the Alexander Graham Bell National Historical Park and Museum near the town of Baddeck. The enormous variety of Mr. Bell's interests and inventions surprised us, and we thoroughly enjoyed the exhibits and history that we learned there. The only fly in the ointment was the boorish behavior of one woman from Quebec, who, intent on what she was viewing jostled us and moved directly in front us, although we had been there before she came along. This was the only disagreeable incident of the whole trip, but made us wonder about how prevalent this sense of entitlement may be among the Quebecois, since we had heard of their rudeness before.

After the museum, we traveled west and south through the rest of Nova Scotia to Peggy's Cove. It is a picturesque little fishing village, which my bridesmaid, Pam had found intriguing for its rustic small fishing port scenes. We enjoyed the views and took a number of photos there. I wanted to buy some touristy items to help remember the trip and tried to use my VISA card in a machine to get money but it wouldn't deliver US dollars; only Canadian. I should have expected that, but was surprised anyway. Dave had wanted to visit the Bay of Fundy to see its famous forty foot tides, but time was catching up with us, so we decided to start home.

The rest of the trip was uneventful, but we marveled at how pleasant the trip had been despite frequent cloudy and drizzly weather which occurred mostly while in the van or sleeping. There had been just enough sun to provide a number of beautiful scenes and to keep us almost entirely dry. We had a great time. On the way home we speculated about the discussions which we thought were going on about us, between Dave's four children. He sent letters as we started our trip, telling them of our marriage and honeymoon. You can imagine our surprise to find that we were not the topic of conversation, which, instead, had been about his youngest son being jailed for driving while impaired during our absence.

The celebration of our marriage was held at the home of Dave's middle son and was attended by Dave's sons, their families and our local friends. It was a delayed wedding reception with me in my wedding dress, the gifts, the wedding cake, tossing of the garter, etc. When we cut the cake, I had fun smearing a piece of wedding cake on Dave's face and he returned the favor. It was another great time.

Our engagement, wedding, reception and honeymoon had been more of an adventure because of the different order of events. We were engaged for quite awhile, but kept it and the wedding secret until the honeymoon. The honeymoon was delayed several weeks because I was working, and neither of us could get off from work immediately. Instead of an immediate reception, we had the celebration of the marriage several weeks after the honeymoon. I kidded Dave, "You never take me anywhere."

We had wanted to get a dog, but couldn't because our rental wouldn't permit it. As a child, I always wanted a collie, but we never had one. With Dave's and my love of the breed, we started exploring how to obtain an affordable collie, for when we would be able to buy a home. Since full blooded collies are expensive, we went to the local dog shelter, where we found an old collie. Dave called it a salesman, because it gave me one paw, and then another, as it sought an owner. It was a beautiful Lassie type dog, but because of its age, and our not wanting to lose it within the next two to four years; we decided to look some more.

Soon, I saw a breeder's ad in a news paper for collies. I called the breeder about the ad and we went to see her pups and full grown dogs. She obviously loved them, since many had both kennels and the run of the house. One full sized long haired tricolor named Ralph had a healed, previously broken a rear leg. The dog's fine formation and disposition had caused her to want to show it competitively. She was deeply disappointed by the broken leg because even fully healed it made competitive showing impossible. We were in the process of buying our first home, but had not settled yet. We bought the dog, at a reduced price because of the broken leg, and asked the breeder to hold it until the house was settled. She did, and Dave and I went to see Ralph as often as possible for several weeks. With no children and no plans for any, Ralph's loving nature soon changed our thinking of him from a dog to a beloved member of the family. We renamed him Pal.

Pal was more Dave's dog than mine. He was very obedient to him and tried to do whatever Dave wanted. Because he was so dependable in coming when called, he used to walk him without a leash. Later he started to use a leash when he realized, that with the variety of dangers from cars, people and other animals, Pal could be hurt in spite of his dependable obedience. Pal deeply loved me and I loved him, but as far as he was concerned, Dave was Alpha and I was Beta. The one time he became somewhat estranged from us was when Dave and I went on our honeymoon, and Pal was left with our friend Ann. When we returned he seemed confused about his relationship with us. Instead of his usual behavior of being as close to us as possible he lay across the room and seemed sad rather than his usual eager, sunny self. I think it was a case of I don't know where I belong. Why were you gone so long? Why did you leave me? It took Pal a while to get over our absence. Ann took good care of Pal while we were gone, but we didn't get the welcome home that we expected. It wasn't too long before he was again the animal who always was by our side and could be depended upon to be pressed against us whenever we were seated or lying down.

A SCIENTIFIC
ORGANIZATION

I obtained work at a scientific organization. The work was primarily ordering animals for well over a hundred researchers, but included a variety of other administrative duties. It was very time consuming and involved demands for many emergency deliveries, because of poor planning by the researchers. To make matters worse, through no fault of the researchers, many orders had to be planned well in advance. This was because the condition of the ordered animals was time sensitive, either due to the need to be in a particular condition, or because of the rarity of particular animals. I reduced the constant emergency orders by insisting on justification for each emergency order, which annoyed those researchers, who found advance planning difficult (for which I wasn't to be forgiven by some).

Other administrative duties involved timekeeping, and ordering general goods and services. Some orders were standard orders, but most were individual, as needed. I reduced emergency orders, by requiring justifications. Another occasional duty was typing of scientific protocols before they went to an animal use and care committee to be approved for each study. These protocols are very strict and specific in requiring maximum consideration for creature safety and comfort possible in the designs of the studies.

My supervisor's style of supervision was based on perfectionism rather than leadership and involved micromanaging. Emphasis was on mistakes in ordering, no matter how small and insignificant the mistakes or whether self corrected without any problems. They were kept on a daily chart, and I was given minimally satisfactory performance evaluations, which tended to discourage promotion or transfer. I was unable to satisfy, despite a substantial number of complementary statements and memos from the scientists about the excellence of my service in the ordering of their animals. They were particularly pleased with my keeping them informed about expected time lapses for delivery of rare animals, because of the time sensitivity of some of their experiments. This was a service, which they had not received dependably from my job predecessor. They also complemented my courtesy and professionalism.

After nearly five years of increasingly unreasonable job pressure, I resigned. The pressure was despite the satisfaction of the vast majority of the many scientists I served. I had come to the conclusion that the unrelenting, unjustified pressure and weak performance ratings (satisfactory at the present time) could not work to my advantage, and I might as well go back to temp assignments, until I could find more satisfactory employment.

DAD'S DEATH

Toward the end of my work at the scientific organization I received word that Dad was very ill. He was living with the woman for whom, he had left Mom. Dave and I drove, on an extended weekend to see him. I discovered that he had cancer and was likely to die. With this in mind I told him that I forgave him and talked to him about believing in Jesus. He was indignant that I thought he needed to be forgiven, and rejected, what he claimed, was worthless religion. A few days later we received word that he had been operated on, and that things seemed better. But this didn't last long; the cancer spread and, before long, he was dead.

My oldest brother, Johan, who I hadn't seen in years, appeared at the burial and we talked. He told me that Dad had used my epilepsy as an excuse to avoid service in the Korean War on the basis of my physical disabilities. I thought, how sweet of him to use my epilepsy to stay out of active danger, where there was the most opportunity for promotion, and blame me for failure to increase in rank. In effect he was claiming that his failure to get promoted was my fault, rather than his own decision to avoid danger, and his poor behavior in destroying bars and not respecting authority. Of course he may have actually been thinking of us in his request.

I'll never know. But, it was good to see Johan, and talk even if only for a little while.

I wish things could have been different between Johan and me. Our relationship was strained after he started having seizures and had a personality change, from loving brother to self consumed jerk, who didn't care who he hurt to get what he wanted or how he got it. Johan liked life in the fast lane and I just wanted to have a normal life. To this day, I still feel angry with Johan's robbing us of a good relationship. I don't understand why things had to go so sour between us. I never saw Johan alive again.

VISITS WITH LAURA

At about five years of age Laura was having a bit of an identity crisis. With remarriage, her mother had a new last name but Laura's last name hadn't changed. This troubled her and she wanted her name to be the same as her step-dad and mother's. This posed a problem, because Phil had not legally given up his parental rights. Since Phil believed he was not yet equipped to be the father Laura deserved he agreed to do so. Laura was adopted by Dan, her step-father, and also went to court to have her name changed. During the early part of this while Laura was still troubled about the name differences Dave and I went to visit her to try and provide some emotional continuity to go with the occasional long distance phone conversations and presents I had been sending. I had been trying to give other kinds of support earlier before Virginia remarried, when she might have been able to use some assistance with Christmas presents and inexpensive clearance clothing as I was able to afford it.

We drove south visiting in their home, where Virginia had moved to take advantage of an opportunity offered by her employer. I had the pleasure of playing for the first time with my niece and meeting Dan. At this age Laura was fascinated with her dolls and wanted me to play with them with her. This was fun as I found her to be charming, bright and articulate for her age. Dan was a keeper. My not having any children or, expecting to have any, made these opportunities more precious. The few days we spent there were a delight and we looked forward to other face to face opportunities. Several years later we were able to arrange, with Virginia and Dan, for Laura to visit us.

Dave and I met her at Dulles airport. They had put her on the plane, arranging for the stewardess to watch out for her. Craft items and some planned activities outside the home entertained her well one day. It gave me pleasure to see her enjoying them. Another day we drove to Baltimore to their great aquarium. It was a delight, with huge tanks that contained many varieties of large and small fish on both sides of the aisles and were observable from the floor above. The dolphin show was the main hit. It had large dolphins doing a number of tricks with a variety of objects and making spectacular leaps out of the water in association with their handlers. One of the males seemed to be horny, swimming rapidly around after females. To the amusement of some of the nearby spectators young Laura wanted to know what was that thing sticking out from the under belly of a dolphin as it flew around in the pool. I told her that she'd have to ask her mother.

The last day she and two of Dave's granddaughters made individual apple pies from scratch as part of a county agricultural activity. It looked marvelous and, having tasted some from samples provided from the same baking batch, I know that the taste was great. However, Laura was intent on taking it home. We heard later that without specialized packing it arrived more like a cobbler but still delicious.

TEMP JOBS

During this period I applied to a number of personnel agencies that recruited and supplied temporary workers and my employment was a series of temporary assignments with several of these companies. This was greatly assisted by my varied office training and experience. In order to maintain almost continuous employment, I continued my practice of learning new office softwares. A marvelous little computer software training school, just a few blocks from our home was especially helpful. They allowed me take a variety of courses, on an affordable, pay as you go, basis. It was here that I learned Excel and Access. They have proven to be particularly useful additions to my office software body of knowledge, and resultant ability to obtain increasingly highly paid assignments.

It was fortunate that I had continued my HMO coverage with a private plan, because my husband, Dave, developed a benign cancer of his left inner ear. Benign cancers are slower growth cancers, which, because of their slow development, are less likely to be fatal. However, they can do considerable damage. This one, called an acoustic neuroma, caused almost complete hearing loss and altered or destroyed balance signals from that inner ear. The immediate result of the balance signal loss was extreme vertigo.

Vertigo happens when the signals to the brain, from an inner ear, which can account for, thirty five to forty per cent of total balance information from each ear, are different from the usual pattern. If the difference is very slight it may produce a little whirling sensation, similar that, of riding a merry-go-round. However, the change of balance signals from his left ear were major and resulted in vomiting and sweating, with the automatic systems in the brain seeming to interpret the differences in signal patterns, from those usually received from other balance sensors, as the result of poisoning. We believe the vomiting and sweating was the body's attempt to rid itself of a possible poison. Also, the signal loss caused enough confusion in the portion of the brain, which interprets balance signals, to disturb the ability to stand, let alone walk. The vertigo persisted for many months as our HMO tried at first to understand what was happening and then find the best treatment solution.

Finally, they decided that they needed to refer us to specialists, at either a famous Washington area hospital or an equally famous hospital forty miles away, in Baltimore. We chose Baltimore, with its brilliant reputation, to do the delicate surgery necessary to reduce or kill the neuroma, and Dave had gamma knife radiation surgery there. They took an impression of his face and used it to create a mold. This was used to bolt his head precisely in an unmovable position for five treatments with gamma rays focused on the neuroma from four hundred different angles. We were told that the neuroma was destroyed though twenty years later a general practitioner claimed that it might still be growing. We believe the surgeons rather than the g.p.

After Dave received the radiation treatment, the vertigo stopped for about a month, before it returned with a vengeance. We were told that the swelling, to the immediate area from the gamma rays, was going down, resulting in variable signals going to the brain again. When the swelling was gone, the vertigo stopped. However, it took months. His vertigo caused me to lose several temp assignments, while staying home to take care of him. It was then, that I learned to drive a car all over again, in order to get home in a hurry to be able to quickly transport him for medical help.

I had not attempted to drive since Dad's failed attempt to teach me so many years earlier, But now I had to try again. My classes were at a cheap little driving school. The classroom work was alright although the rooms were crowded and needed air conditioning. But the driving instruction left a lot to be desired. My instructor barely spoke English and practice was in a filthy car, which had stinky clothing in the back seat. He showed me how to back into a parking space, but not how to correct when I misjudged. Because of this, although the school's certificate of completion allowed me to obtain a learner's permit, I was still unable to back into a parking space dependably in the allotted time. Thus my attempt at the Maryland driving test was a failure. I was allowed to retake the driving part of the test on another day.

Dave was still having vertigo that was somewhat controlled by drugs. Over a weekend, he gave me intensive instruction in parallel parking. This was critical because I had delayed, until the last few days before the scheduled expiration of my learners permit. It was Friday and I had to pass the test on Monday or reapply for a permit all over again after a required period of delay. I spent almost the entire weekend practicing reverse parking to the point that I had aching muscles. It worked; I passed and, now, can park more efficiently than Dave.

It would be nice if I could report that this was the end of my driver license problems. My slowness in completing the requirements of the permit only allowed me to get a restricted license, newly more rigorous as required by law. This was designed to better prepare drivers for a full license. It required, forty hours of driving to be supervised and reported on specific aspects as outlined in a booklet supplied by the Motor Vehicle Administration (MVA) and that all of my driving for eighteen months be accompanied by a licensed driver. As if that wasn't enough, my epilepsy, which we hadn't hidden from MVA, caused them to insist on a medical assurance from my neurologist that my seizures had been under control for an extended period. Also, they ran my record through their own medical board, and insisted on my taking their brake reaction test. I took the test while they held my license and found the wait for the results excruciating, not knowing, if after all this, I would be allowed to drive. Finally the tester returned and gave me back my license back. Of course we notified our auto insurer of these developments

I had been a snorer since childhood but Dave had become alarmed, because I seemed to stop breathing for stretches before snorting and starting to breathe again. He kept pestering me to have this checked. Also during this time, with the lack of enough rest, I fell asleep on jury duty. This was an embarrassment to me and the prosecutor was not too pleased, nearly removing me from the jury. But with some caffeinated beverages I was able to stay awake and complete my service. Finally I decided to do something about it. My HMO doctor said that I might have obstructive sleep apnea and recommended a study in a sleep study lab. This involved spending the night in the lab monitored by equipment and personnel. Since Dave was snoring too we decided to do the study together. After the test they said that I woke everyone up during it. More importantly they reported that I had failed to breathe, while sleeping, for periods of between nineteen and twenty-nine seconds and the problem was a severe case of obstructed sleep apnea which could be improved by using a CPap machine. This blows air up the nose to overcome the obstruction which appears with the relaxation of sleep. My HMO paid for half the price of the machine. Dave's apnea was less severe and didn't require any equipment.

Several years after the killing of the acoustic neuroma cancer, Dave started having vertigo again. We wondered if the cancer had returned, and our doctors did a lot of testing, but couldn't provide a clear diagnosis. The doctors were treating the symptoms, since this was the safest procedure without a clear diagnosis and with the possibility that the cancer might have returned. The treatment was Phenergan pills, to stop the nausea, and did nothing to identify the problem or attack it.

The vertigo caused nausea, violent vomiting and the sweating all over again. I remember several times, when Dave called me from the kitchen, to bring him a waste basket, because he was starting to spew. He needed to get to the living room, to lie down on the couch until it stopped. I brought him a waste basket and folded a sheet on the couch to soak up perspiration. This was so he could crawl through the dining room to the couch, with my holding the waste basket under his head for the gush. The pills had to stay down to be effective, but were coming back up. I phoned the doctors to find out how to proceed. They said that I should give him Phenergan as a suppository and gave me a prescription. So I learned to administer suppositories.

Since we had great success with treating the neuroma at the hospital in Baltimore, I insisted on working with them again to solve this new vertigo problem. Finally, after a lot of nagging, our HMO approved working with a wonderfully world renowned doctor there. After a series of tests at his vestibular laboratory, he determined that Dave had Menier's like symptoms, probably somewhat modified by damage to surrounding tissue, by the gamma knife radiation treatments, used to kill the cancer several years earlier. Until this time the only treatment was to reduce the vomiting, not attack the unknown underlying problem. Now, he prescribed a drastic reduction of salt in diet and several specific medicines to try to treat the problem. With these standard procedures for Menier's in place, as these drugs were tried, the second one began to control the vertigo. Finally, after a year or more, it disappeared entirely, even with the complete, but gradual weaning off the medicines.

An interesting side note happened a few months before Dave's referral and the diagnosis of Menier's like symptoms. His dentist, of all people, told him that although Menier's was not curable, he had read in the literature that something, possibly a virus, was appearing that mimicked Menier's. This entity appeared to run its course in two or three years. Because of the length of time the new medical procedure took to cure the vertigo, it appears that Dave's condition may have been caused by that mysterious entity, made more difficult to diagnose, by damage from the gamma knife treatment, as our doctor surmised.

A BLIND SUPPORT
ORGANIZATION

Finally, all the software training and experience began to pay off in permanent employment, with an interesting job as administrative assistant/office manager to the director of a nonprofit organization which supported the blind. This organization taught people losing their sight or, already blind, how to adapt to blindness with a variety of programs, from use of a cane, for walking about independently, to using other methods, strategies and tools to substitute for sight. It supplied many of these tools through a small store that sold canes, talking clocks, talking telephones, etc. at modest prices. It also furnished, blindness compatible, computer software and job training in M S Word to help clients make themselves economically self sufficient through clerical work.

The company's director and most of the employees were blind. I read them their telephone messages or had a sighted co-worker type them in Braille. Careful communication was very important in order to bridge the differences from sightedness to blindness. I soon realized that this disability, while in many ways devastating, can, never-the-less, be overrated. The blind can be very independent and do many things, at least as well, and sometimes better than many sighted people, when they have adopted the necessary strategies, methods and tools.

As the Office Manager I made certain that things ran smoothly in the office. This was much more than the usual range of activity, because I frequently acted as the eyes of the director. I also learned a few elements of Braille in order to perform Braille related duties, and backed up the company accountant to make sure that bills were paid in the accountant's absence.

I was asked to help train our students in basic computer software and MS Word for office work. In order to do this, I had to relearn DOS, because Windows is not compatible with blindness. I taught them DOS and, in MS Word, to create labels and merge letters, etc. It was personally rewarding to watch my students learn, knowing that I was helping them be more independent, and equipped for gainful employment.

One of my blind students was the managing director of a small local theater company. He needed a database of information to be used in a variety of ways by his organization. Its main proposed uses seemed to be for communicating with members and interested parties about solicitations, announcements, directions, etcetera. It needed to be broken down by geographic areas and to list enough personal data to optimize usefulness of the information to involve the people in the database in the company's programs if they had an interest in being active participants. This was beyond the scope of activities of the blind organization, but I had just completed a course in the computer program called ACCESS.

It is difficult to design a database with ACCESS because of the large variety of details necessary to be planned, in the beginning, to accommodate its many possible uses. The problem is that, once the basic categories are set, it has to be limited to those planned units. It is too late to add other information categories once the plan is set and the data is being entered. But, with careful anticipation of uses and setup, to cover all needed data, it is very easy to use. It saves huge amounts of time in communicating with those, in the database. I wanted to practice ACCESS and was intrigued at the chance to be a major participant in the expansion of the theater company. Design of the database was volunteered personal time but I didn't have time to maintain it. Several years later I heard that the database had fifty thousand individuals. It made a nice addition to my resume and involved me actively in this aspect of theater management for a little while.

Though new students often felt that their situations were hopeless, they weren't. They had counselors to help them learn how to walk properly with a cane, to operate computer software, to read Braille and many other necessary adaptations. It was a pleasure working there and serving the blind community, but was not without its problems. The director seemed to be very angry at being blind and to take it out on sighted persons. She seemed to think that all of them intended to cheat the blind and may have had some very bad experiences with cheats. For example, cheating in the exchange of money can be a fairly common problem for the blind. But it is not necessarily the rule. Since it is attempted from time to time, it is necessary for blind persons to be wary in the exchange of money and to learn methods to distinguish between denominations of bills by tactics such as positioning different denominations in their own locations in wallets, or by folding them in special ways and to keep enough bills and variety in bills to be able to make proper change. But, other than making blind people or people losing their sight, aware that they will run into some cheats, and providing defensive tactics, it isn't helpful to communicate an overall attitude of anger against sighted people.

Also I had a major problem upon discovering that reports required for funding from several major donor organizations were seriously in arrears. When I pointed this out to the director nothing was done to correct this problem. Since this endangered the viability of the organization, I reported it to the board of directors. Finally I decided that I couldn't be part of management that was this ragged and resigned. A year or so later the organization went out of business.

About this time our faithful collie, Pal had begun to slow down and seemed to have trouble with his hind legs. He wasn't able to play hide and seek on the first floor of the house any more. He couldn't go with me on walks and be my growling protector, he had been, on the few times he had felt it necessary. We believed the problem was old age and, because collies as a breed have a reputation for epilepsy, we wondered if he might have it. It was not to be, but what he had was just as serious. A few weeks after recognizing his increasing difficulty with his legs I was awakened by a noise and discovered Pal sprawled out at the bottom of the stairs. He couldn't stand up, so we stayed with him, gently rubbing his head, neck and shoulders to comfort him until we could contact our veterinarian. He told us to bring him to his office immediately. Pal was a full sized collie so it wasn't easy to haul him to the car seventy yards down the courtyard in comfort without dropping him. But we did it, with my comforting him on the back seat, until we arrived. The vet said to go home, that he had to do some diagnostics and would phone us with the results. In early afternoon he reported that Pal had a cancer in the part of the brain that controls the legs. He also had several seizures while there, and that he would have to be put down. When Dave went to pick up his body the vet said that Pal had been so good natured that he went out of his way to be with him while researching the problem and that he had administered sedative to allow him to had die peacefully. Dave buried him in the black plastic bag in which the vet had placed him. Pal was so beloved in the neighborhood that our neighbor, seven houses away at the other end of the courtyard, insisted on helping dig the grave. It was at least five feet deep and they put the sod back over it leaving bare ground a few feet away in case any curious or mischievous neighbors decided to dig him up while we were both at work.

I was broken up at losing my good buddy, who was such a loving dog, always wanting to be right next to Dave or me. An immediate search for a replacement collie located a four year old in a collie rescue organization in a rural area a few miles up county. It had belonged to woman in northern Virginia who was forced to give him up because she was moving to an apartment that didn't allow large dogs. We obtained Chester within three days of Pal's death. His markings were so similar that a number of the neighbors thought he was Pal until we told them what had happened. He was another fine dog but with a slightly different personality. Pal was the ultimate love dog, always desiring to please but Chester specialized in play.

He enriched our live for about seven years. While Pal had been Dave's dog, Chester was mostly mine possibly because I took more time to play with him. Near the end of his time with us we didn't know what was wrong with him, so we took him to the vet. She stated that Chester had a fever and his lymph nodes were very swollen. She did a fine needle aspiration but didn't see anything, so, she sent the cells to the lab for further examination. The results came back that Chester had Cancer of the Lymph Nodes. He was another great collie. a true champ, never complaining and I have no regret in getting him after Pal died. Chester usually made me feel better about myself since he made no demands and loved to play hide-&-seek, playing more skillfully than Pal. By the time he was 13 years old with a tired body; he didn't always want to play. But when he did I would play our game of hide and seek and he usually found me. His not being able to climb the steps to go to bed with us was upsetting but he knew he was loved. He died at a local animal care organization. I believe collies are the best dogs. They are sensitive, caring and obedient. They want their entire pack together and HAPPY!! Chester also wanted to please but his main interest was play and to be always at my side.

A SCIENTIFIC
LABORATORY

I started working for a temporary service providing personnel to a scientific laboratory. The job was working for the director of the laboratory, which involved the entire campus of approximately forty scientists and sometimes the other twenty scientists who worked for him at another location. When interviewed for the job, I was asked what I could do. I said it depended on what was needed and was told to create an office.

The previous secretary worked there for many years and had become ill with narcolepsy. As the illness developed, she found keeping awake increasingly difficult and tried to use the caffeine of coffee and sodas to stay awake, but nothing worked dependably. Spilled beverages had made her computer keyboard inoperable and glued the monitor to the desk. Toward the end of her work there, she had brought in blankets and a pillow, to sleep during lunch. In her constantly sleepy condition, she had become very inefficient, so that the office was in complete chaos. It stank and there were as many as twenty years of old documents in disarray, much of it items, which should have been distributed to employees. The director was a very compassionate man, and had overlooked this until the situation had become impossible.

He instructed me to throw out all paper which was over five years old, except for scientific periodicals and treatises, needed to establish a small library. After throwing out barrels of trash, I sorted the remaining documents and set up filing systems. This was a huge effort, taking many weeks, just to arrange and file the basic systems of the office. The organizing was happening while taking on an increasing routine of current activity. The library had to be organized as the daily responsibilities would allow, which made it take much longer. Organizing the office was not a onetime thing, but rather involved trial and error of systems to find the optimal arrangements. Gradually, I created a smoothly running office that relieved administrative pressures on the director, as he assigned me a steadily increasing number and variety of duties. In time, I became his administrative assistant and point of contact for people needing to deal with the lab in administrative functions. After about a year, my employment status was changed from a temporary to a contract employee in providing services in holiday, annual leave and sick leave benefits to the lab's employees.

While organizing the office and acquiring added duties I was taking training in making travel arrangements. Travel preparation out of the country was sufficiently different that training was presented in two courses. Continuing office organizing, doing the personnel paperwork and learning the two courses, which were presented almost simultaneously, was too much all at once. The administrative officer, who was responsible for the director's budget and my training in travel planning, decided that I was too slow in learning travel planning. She reduced my travel planning responsibilities for awhile. This was accompanied by a reduction of my work week from forty to thirty hours and an equivalent loss in pay. The reduced cost to the budget could have been the main motive for the reduction of my work hours. The activity was soon restored but the paid hours never were. The reduced hours endangered my health insurance benefits, if my hours were cut any further.

Later, when another travel planner at the other campus took a several month extended leave of absence, I planned the travel of his approximately twenty scientists who worked there, in another group, responsible to the director, (The only time I had any responsibility for them). This was without any increase in my thirty weekly paid hours and despite the fact that I worked over fifty hours a week to be sure that the scientists' travel documents were prepared and paid in timely fashion. I volunteered the extra time because of my appreciation for the way I was being encouraged and allowed to grow professionally from the time I started working for him. I'm proud of the fact that my office organizing produced a system more efficient for finding documents than the office of the administrative officer who was supposed to have general responsibility for administrative functions at our lab. From time to time, they had to phone and ask that materials they had already received be refaxed because of inability to find them in their files which were less meticulously organized. Another source of personal satisfaction comes from the fact that the director resisted attempts by them to change my systems, after I left, because mine were so efficient and easy to use.

The laboratory did much of its research on monkeys, investigating their behaviors in many different situations and stages of their lives. This is because relatively simple lab situations can be arranged relatively easily and clearly to obtain information about how variations of factors produce behavior and development.

In our very complex human situations, it is much more difficult to identify, which of the many factors is influencing what result, and to what degree. Also, we would not be allowed to arrange human environment to the degree that we can for monkeys. These simpler situations yield valuable clues about what strategies are useful in teaching and encouraging optimum human development and motivation. The established and emerging results have many applications and are of wide interest. These scientists present their findings to their professional associations, related scientific groups, education and motivation researchers, and are invited to many symposia and conferences, at the inviting organization's expense. The director constantly has his new scientific findings published, and his several hundred articles are so popular that he attended thirty to forty of these functions annually, frequently as the keynote speaker. These presentations took him all over the country and the world usually at the expense of the inviting organization. He could have attended many more, if time and work had permitted.

A major part of my work involved arranging, for the laboratory and the inviting organizations, the details of travel to his and our other scientists' functions, as the travel planner. It meant contact with people, wherever travel was to be scheduled, and was especially interesting when it involved foreign countries. I arranged travel, lodging, per diem, and who would pay for what, in written agreements so that everything would be clear and establish responsibilities between the various entities in line with established arrangements. The most difficult and interesting involved presentations in different countries with as many as four different stops in one long business trip.

I enjoyed all of this activity, because of the contacts, but especially because the director encouraged me to work with considerable independence, to organize and make continuing change to the office as needed. He didn't want to be bothered with any more administrative details, than absolutely necessary and took my suggestions seriously. He allowed recommendations about needed equipment, which he often let me select. He was open to new ideas, generally a fair and an excellent supervisor, the best I have had, as of the writing of this book. Working with him, was by far the most productive work that I have performed. It filled me with confidence in my abilities, as well as provided a huge jump in the responsibilities of the jobs that I applied for and obtained. This has been reflected in my earnings at most of these positions.

After the return of the other travel planner from several months extended leave, I stopped planning the travel of his twenty scientists. One of them had especially appreciated my informing him of legitimate travel entitlements that the other planner should have told him about. To show his appreciation, he brought me a souvenir cup, from the trip that I planned, to Paris, France. It felt good, to receive his and other scientists' thanks for the thoroughness and quality of my work. But I would have appreciated being paid, at least, forty hours weekly, of the over fifty hours necessary to plan the travel of the extra twenty scientists for the several months of the other planner's leave.

I felt justified in requesting a little vacation. Dave and I took a whirlwind scenic drive across country and back in just a little over a week in our new automobile. We drove west, out of the Washington metropolitan area, on interstate route 66(I66) toward I81, which goes southwest into the northeastern corner of Tennessee. A few hours after crossing the border on I81 we drove onto I40 a little east of Knoxville. It took us through the musical cities of Nashville and Memphis, famous for country music and Elvis Pressley.

Our first destination was Fort Smith, Arkansas, on the Oklahoma border, to visit Dave's friend and former associate. He took us out to dinner and put us up for the night in his parents' lovely home. He was house sitting, while they were vacationing in Europe. We slept in the huge guest room, our fanciest accommodations of the trip, and Dave's friend played chef for breakfast the next morning. Then it was west on I40, across Oklahoma and north Texas to New Mexico

We paused in Gallop to look at some Indian memorials, eat, and shop at a store selling Indian crafts and memorabilia. The restaurant was different; Indians came to our table selling small craft items, colorful earthenware mugs, jewelry, etc. When we left the restaurant, a man who looked like an Indian, said that I had better leave; that he hated me. That gave me something to think about. At a nearby store we found many colorful traditional Indian items for sale, head dresses, bows and arrows, woven goods, stoneware, etc.

Then we went into Arizona, and off of I40, southwest toward the Phoenix suburb of Mesa, where Mom is buried. Several months earlier, we had finally purchased a headstone for Mom's grave, and the cemetery had promised to try to install it before our arrival. There it was, under the tree that I had requested for her grave site. I liked the stone and was pleased to see how peaceful and well kept everything looked. Mesa is special to me for Mom's grave. The cemetery management kept the gravesite clean with fresh flowers on it. I had forgotten how kind these people were after Mom died. When she died, I think a part of me died; I was alone without my partner, my best friend. I still miss her so much!!

After perhaps an hour, we headed north toward Sedona. We had heard that it was very beautiful. It didn't disappoint us, as we stopped along the road to take photos of the buttes, cliffs and colorful rock formations. We found it so enchanting that we decided to try and photograph it from the air, arriving at a local air tour company just in time to fly over Sedona's valleys and canyons at sunset. It was gorgeous and we were able to get lots of pictures from the small high winged plane. Knowing that we were trying to squeeze a lot of sightseeing into a short trip, we drove until very late, and finally located a motel fairly near the Grand Canyon

The next morning we got up early and, after breakfast, drove to the south rim of the canyon. We spent the next few hours traveling from one part of the south rim to another, enjoying the marvelous views. It was sunny, and the sunlight on the varied colored rock formations as far as the eye could see, won't be forgotten. Its size is immense, one mile straight down, if you could go straight down, is so much more than you can imagine that it is impossible to be disappointed. This would have made an even better place to take an airplane tour than Sedona, but, with the immensity of it, would have been even more expensive. We were beginning to limit our expenses, but that didn't prevent me from buying trinkets, DVDs, and photographic murals of this incredible place.

Dave told me that on a previous visit with a friend, they were standing on the south rim in falling snow, in upper thirty degree weather, talking to another family. These folks said that their children and grand children were down in the bottom of the canyon, and that, on the previous day, were in over hundred degree weather. We continued driving from one good view on the south rim to another. Walking good distances to get to some of the best viewing points was tiring, and we had many other wonderful places to see in our quick trip, so we regretfully shortened our visit there. It was a particularly memorable part of the trip; our special time. It was so much more than what I had expected: the colors, the canyons, the telescopes, the animals and of course, the beauty of the land. Just breathtaking!! We only viewed from a part of the south rim and will want to visit the Canyon again, with more time to enjoy its many attractions.

I wanted to go to Las Vegas next, but, Dave, with his dislike of gambling, reminded me that our emphasis of the trip was scenic beauty, and that we still had a lot of travel to squeeze into a little time. So, after going south to I40, we continued west, well south of Vegas through the Mohave Desert in California on I40 to near Barstow where we switched to California route 58. It was somewhere along here that I was driving through an unlit tunnel without my eyes having adjusted to the darkness. I told Dave that I was going to stop because; I was having trouble seeing the road. There were cars behind us, and he said, "No, you're not, because of them." I was afraid and angry, but slowed down and did as he said. When we left the tunnel, I pulled to the side to calm down. The following drivers zoomed past, with the first one flashing the famous finger.

I remember lunch in Bakersfield; then it was more westward travel on 58. As the afternoon wore on we drove down out of the mountains, and saw the sun displaying the tops of the puffy white clouds ahead of us, and then down through the grey fog that clouds look like from the inside. We stayed on 58 until it ended a little east of the famously beautiful coastal route 1. By then, it was night, but we kept going. In the small town, Cayucos, we found a colorful little motel with a marvelous flower garden backyard, and its view of the Pacific Ocean. Each room was decorated with a different marine motif. It was modest but comfortable and the sea scenes on the walls and other marine decorations provide a pleasant memory. They reduced the price because we arrived so late and were leaving the next day, which made it even more memorable. They said that they had our room booked immediately after we were due to leave and that they had many bookings by people, who requested the same rooms they had occupied before, on honeymoons and other special occasions.

The next morning, after breakfast and viewing the garden with the ocean view, we started north along scenic route 1. Our lunch was in Cambria a neat and clean town which seemed rather upscale and pricey to us. The food was good, but expensive, as was the gasoline. The entire route 1 from the south end, north of San Luis Obispo to San Francisco has major stretches of road either in view of the Pacific Ocean or practically above the beach looking down on it. On one of these spots we got out to enjoy the wild flowers and the walruses sleeping on the beach. The vistas of waves splashing on rocky shores interspersed with little beaches on the left and a variety of hilly scenes on the right helped make this a spiritually uplifting drive.

We had talked about seeing Big Sur and the wonders of Monterey Bay. Unfortunately, we hadn't researched the area enough and drove on by before we fully realized it. With our emphasis on seeing Yosemite National Park, and other natural beauty in the little time that we had left, we decided not to go back on roads that weren't familiar but possibly visit them another time.

So it was on to San Francisco where I wanted to be sure to see Chinatown and to ride the cable cars, which I liked to call the Rice-A-Roni cable cars after a popular advertising on T V. Our first problem in San Francisco was to find inexpensive lodging for the night since it was getting late in the day. A few questions to some locals provided suggestions to check the area around the zoo. We found a somewhat run down motel that seemed pricy, but I insisted on staying there for the night rather than looking further. The next morning I was all set to ride my Rice-A-Roni cars and to see China town. We were very impressed with the steepness of the hilly streets but, once again, had not researched. Driving around looking for both attractions, we drove through China town but didn't find a place to park. We didn't know where the cable cars were or where to park our car if we found them. The cost of a very ordinary motel, along with not knowing our way around, soured our attitude toward San Francisco.

Eager to get to Yosemite, we drove east across the Bay Bridge on US80 to Oakland and south on US580 which turned east below San Leandro. After about forty seven miles from starting U580 back in Oakland, we continued east on US205 about thirteen miles to a somewhat northward swing on US5 to where route 120 goes east. We proceeded on 120 fifty six miles through increasingly rural country to go south on route 49 eighteen miles to a rustic restaurant in Coulterville where we ate a late lunch. We didn't find the food particularly memorable but enjoyed the old time décor of the rough wood exterior and interior paneling along with a few pieces of small old fashioned farm equipment as decorations. Not having seen any motels for a number of miles through this rural area we continued south on route 49 until we spotted an interesting looking motel up a hill on the left perhaps ten or twelve miles south of Coulterville. It was a little early to choose a motel but too late to drive into Yosemite and hope to find lodging in such a popular place. With this in mind we decided to check it out.

This was not a five star establishment, but seemed neat and clean looking and, with its location high up on the hill, had a nice view. Also, the exterior had some pleasant tree plantings around an informal patio with some wooden tables and chairs in an area loosely fenced in with a split rail fence. I seem to remember a few plastic outdoor toys such as small tricycles in that area also. We pulled in, registered, and I started snapping pictures of the area. The interior was pleasant but unremarkable and we don't even remember if they had dining. But it was clean, comfortable, inexpensive and reasonably close to Yosemite National Park. It was pleasant and very well fit our needs for a place to stay near the park.

The next day it was off to Yosemite. This was not the best year to visit, because on the way to the office, there were areas, as far as you could see, apparently burned by forest fire. The vistas were of large numbers of charred leafless tree skeletons sitting on equally burned ground. However, after we passed that, we drove over a small one or two lane bridge with a little water fall/rapids on the left. After snapping a few pictures we moved on toward the huge parking area and offices of the park. It has been long enough that we can't provide an accurate narrative but can tell of some that caught our attention. I took a few snapshots of the lovely little creek running through the park with the sunlight threading through the trees on the rippling water, shoreline and rocks. If I remember correctly, it was at one location along the creek we looked up and saw the mighty boulder, known as El Capitan, famously photographed in black and white by Ansel Adams, the great nature photographer/naturalist who deeply loved Yosemite and hugely influenced both photography and the expansion of the national park system in America. Naturally I had to photograph that. Perhaps the park's most famous example of natural beauty is the exquisite long thin nearly straight down waterfall, known the world over, as Bridal Veil. I took pictures of that from several angles. The park was crowded, as it usually is, but with our planned visit to my relative, who lives near Lake

Tahoe, we decided to leave with only this slight glance at a few of its treasures.

The plan had been to drive east through Yosemite to reach highway 395, shown on the map as a major route north to Lake Tahoe, but the east/west roads through the park were closed by impassable snow. So we drove west on 120 toward routes that would take us toward route 50 that goes east and north around the southeast side of the lake. We no longer remember the exact route (It was most likely 4 or 88 that flow into 395). However, we do remember passing through some beautiful vistas on the right of trees framing distant lakes and snow capped mountains. When we arrived in Nevada on 395 perhaps thirty miles east of Tahoe we stopped in a gas station to phone my relative about our imminent arrival. The call produced the information that this wouldn't be a good time to visit. We were disappointed, but I took the opportunity to put a quarter in a slot machine at the gas station and lost it. Easy come, easy go. So we headed north until we found a motel for the night in a little town where I took a few pictures of the distant mountains in the west.

The following morning it was north on 395 toward route 50 which, after about fifty miles, joins the east/west I80. Somewhere in this area we stopped for breakfast. We weren't looking for anything spectacular, just something simple. This town had a small gas station with an adjoining private restaurant. Our simple breakfast turned into one of the more memorable occasions of the trip. The chef and his wife were new to this location. They had emigrated from Australia a year or so earlier. The place was empty except for ourselves and they had time to schmoose with us. They talked us into an Aussie breakfast. I can't remember what it was, but it was delicious. Moreover, chatting with them about their experiences getting set up and their dreams was one the fun times of the trip. Of the rest of Nevada we remember a series of long salt flats in the brilliant sunlight with low mountains in the distance.

We drove on I80 into Utah past Salt Lake into the beautiful basin, rimmed by snow capped mountains that surround Salt Lake City. By this time it was evening and we found a motel for the night. We had talked about visiting Arches National Park, but our map showed it two hundred thirty eight miles south by southeast of Salt Lake City. I wanted to visit Mount Rushmore, which due is east on I80and north into South Dakota. So we decided that Arches would be too much out of the way and proceeded east the next morning on I80.

Before long we went into Wyoming, where we encountered a snow storm that kept getting heavier as we drove along. I80 was being repaired in long stretches, and the snow was obscuring road markers, so that it was difficult to stay on the part of the road that was drivable. At least in the heavily falling snow we had the road nearly to ourselves. We drove all the way into Laramie and found a pleasant little motel for the night. Waking the next morning revealed that the snow had stopped, but put into question the wisdom of visiting Mount Rushmore on secondary roads under these driving conditions. We chose to continue to Cheyenne and then decide what to do. At Cheyenne it was still very snow covered, so we decided to go south on I25 to Denver, Colorado and east on I70 toward home. By now we were pretty tired, had seen parts of most of the places we wanted to visit and were getting anxious to return home. We continued on I70 all the way through until it reached I270 at Frederick, Maryland and on home.

Sometime after the cross country vacation, I was driving home from work on narrow double lane road, following an eighteen wheel tanker tractor trailer. When I approached another narrow crossroad, to make a right turn, I noticed that the tractor driver was as far to the left as he could get at the intersection ahead of me. His right turn signal was flashing although; I could not see it for the sun shining in my eyes. As a relatively new driver, I associated being on the left automatically with a left turn, not considering that such a large rig would have to turn very wide to make it in a narrow intersection.

I drove up beside the rig on its right side to turn right. As I did, the tanker driver, who couldn't see me in his side mirror, because he had already slightly turned the cab to make the right turn, started his turn. The moving trailer brushed my new car forward, and to the right against a raised berm of earth on the right side of the road. The door glass to my left, shattered into many small pieces, as the metal shrieked, from the pressure of the trailer brushing against the side of the car. I was covered with glass bits, and unnerved by the accident, but couldn't get out of the car, because the berm of earth was holding the right side doors closed, while the trailer was against the left. The tractor driver immediately got out and asked if was alright. I was upset, with no significant cuts or bruises, but had some back strain.

The driver phoned for the police and, when the officer arrived he wrote me a ticket, as the driver responsible for the accident. In fact he looked at what he had written, signed and wrote me another because he said he had forgotten something. Each ticket carried a fine of seventy five dollars and assessed two points against my license. He said that I could appeal the tickets to the court.

It took awhile for the police to cut part of the car to get me out. They put me in an ambulance, and had me taken to the hospital. After I got to there, I kept me waiting and waiting for something, anything to happen. I felt too unnerved to stay and didn't believe anything was broken, so I had Dave drive me home.

I was stiff and sore which was taken care of by my wonderful Chiropractor. I had totaled our car, which meant we would need a new one. It was a hard way to get rid of a car, but I never did like that car!!

I disliked the car, because it had a series of manufacturing or design imperfections, which had to be repaired. As a result although less than happy about the accident I didn't feel terribly badly about the car's loss. We had found earlier, while considering trading it in, that this model had very little resale value and were worried about what the insurance would pay for our totaled vehicle. It was our only car and we would need as much money as possible to help us buy another. To our surprise the insurance company paid us much more than the auto dealers had been willing to offer in trade before the accident. We were determined to get more dependable transportation, and purchased a barely used Toyota Corolla which has served us very well.

When at court to contest the tickets the judge said, that I would have to give the performance of a lifetime to dispute them. I admitted responsibility, but claimed that as a relatively new driver I felt that the penalties for the two tickets were excessive. He agreed and assigned me a fine of $75.00 instead, along with court costs, and suspended the points against my license, provided that I take a renewal course in driving. I took the course and that took care of that.

Gradually, my job at the lab had taken on more duties. I had become timekeeper, keeper of the director's personal credit card, organization credit card (for travel) and of the labs credit card. I certified payroll, created/maintained personnel records, tracked due dates for pay increases and renewal of contracts, and prepared the needed paperwork. I was the point of contact for most non-purely scientific activities of the lab. It had developed into an important job which involved me in many more activities than would have been possible probably anywhere else.

The budget problems continued, and the director's collegial style of management, combined with a severe procrastination problem for administrative details that he appeared to find extremely distasteful, caused him to have considerable conflict with the administrative officer. She appeared to me to overstep her authority occasionally in asking me to give her the number of the director's or lab's organization's credit cards so that she could charge things that she felt were justified. While her motives seemed to be pure, I was unable to do that because the director had told me not to share the card numbers with anyone.

This among other things caused me to fall into disfavor with the administrative officer, who as time went on, harassed me as much as she could. She was unable to get rid of me, because my work was appreciated at the lab, and especially by the director, who wanted as little to do with administration as possible, in order to do his extensive research, writing, and presentations. As a contract employee answerable to him, I was still an employee of the contractor and the administrative officer was the de facto boss of the contractor, so that she was able to pressure him to get at me. Because my relationship with her had deteriorated, I was given mediocre performance ratings and even a warning by the contractor about the need for my conduct to improve. Since I was doing what I had to do and my work was exemplary as far as the lab was concerned, I was caught between the orders of the director, who was my boss and the administrative officer. It was very uncomfortable.

With this in mind, and because I would have better benefits, I decided to seek employment wherever I could find it locally. I recognized that my duties had greatly increased, and varied more widely, than could possibly happened anywhere else. In many other positions, the variety of my duties would have been more compartmentalized between several different specialists. I had no idea how much more qualified this made me and sought jobs well below the value of my new accomplishments.

ALASKA CRUISE

In the fall I decided there was enough annual leave and it was time for another vacation. For a long time, Dave had been interested in Alaska and, gradually, I had come to feel the same especially with the opportunity to take pictures. The pressures of my job and our limited resources restricted the time available for a vacation to about a week. I searched the internet for the cheapest prices, and found that booking in December, for the next summer season would greatly reduce prices for cruises and air fares. We discussed it and bought a one week vacation, a flight to Seattle, overnight Seattle hotel, cruise to Alaska and back, via the inside passage, and flight home. As a Christmas present I bought him a complicated minicam, with the thought that we could use it on our trips, and to record family occasions. This increased my interest even more as I envisioned the opportunity to use it on the trip.

We flew from Dulles International Airport, arriving, at our Seattle hotel about eleven p m for our overnight. This was the only disappointing arrangement of the entire trip. The hotel tried to add extra charges for things which are often customary. They wanted extra for parking, but we had no car, extra for television, and extra to use the phone. We said no to parking and no to t.v., since it was already eleven p.m. and we wanted to get out early in the morning. We also refused the phone service since we didn't plan to phone anyone. Imagine our surprise when we tried to call the hotel's front desk to find no dial tone. No problem; we used my cell phone, but it was stupid, not being able to use their phone to call their front desk. Their internet price, which didn't seem very cheap to us, was obviously a come on. We won't stay there again!

The ship was scheduled to depart the next morning, and we had to be onboard by 10:00 a m. This left us time to get breakfast and wander around the immediate area. We woke about seven, and went looking for a restaurant. It was good exercise, since the area was quite hilly, but we were surprised at the number of restaurants, not yet open. After breakfast and returning to the hotel, we phoned for a cab to take us to the ship. After waiting about twenty minutes for the cab a limousine arrived. The cab was ten minutes late; so after waiting another ten minutes, we decided to splurge on the limo. To our surprise, it didn't seem much more expensive, than what we expected to pay for the cab. I enjoyed the ride in the limo. It was cool having darkened windows so that no one could see us although we could see out.

The huge ship of a major cruise operator, presented a number of new experiences, including obtaining our cruise identification/charge cards, getting the luggage to our room, and selecting the side excursions. Because I had a history of seasickness on ships, I obtained more Dramamine than they routinely issued. Soon we departed Seattle and had lunch in one of the dining rooms. I was thankful, that with the Dramamine, my only difficulty was a little drowsiness. It was a beautifully mild day, and before long, we were in the less crowded waters of Canada's Inside Passage. We cruised all day, passing many beautiful vistas of evergreens, reaching down to the water. Occasionally, we saw light houses and also a few lovely cabins, possibly vacation homes, in these exquisite settings. We waved to the occupants and sometimes they waved back. It was during this first day of cruising, toward Ketchikan, Alaska, that we saw dolphins seemingly racing the ship. They were in and out of sight so quickly that we were unable to photograph them. It was about this time that we discovered Dave should have studied and practiced with his new minicam more because he just barely knew how to operate it.

We arrived at Ketchikan the next morning. It was a quaint little port, bustling with activity near the end of the tourist season. We took a local excursion from a nearby fishing camp, riding in a smaller boat to look for whales and other marine wildlife. It was here that we saw our first humpback whale, and a beach of emperor seals at their rookery. The largest of the seals, called beach masters, kept braying at one another to warn their rivals away from their harems. The crowd of seals on the beach extended into the water, which was so crowded that it seemed almost all fins, bodies and splashes. Returning to camp, we saw a bald eagle in a treetop, a red fox on the beach and a little waterfall on a sharp hill next to the camp. Naturally, I was snapping pictures the whole time and Dave was trying to use the minicam with very limited success.

Upon our return to the center of town we visited some of the shops and bought souvenirs. We looked for a seafood place to buy and ship fresh salmon. Since it was expensive to buy and ship frozen, so we settled for dried, bought some for ourselves and for Dave's oldest son and his family. Each port visit was long enough to tour, shop and eat out, although sumptuous fare was always available on board at meal times and lighter fare all day long. Nights were spent on board, cruising to the next scheduled port.

Next was Tracy Arm of the Inside Passage, with its own glacier. We cruised up to it to view from the ship, but our ship was so huge that we couldn't get close. Never-the-less the sight was awe inspiring. It was here, that we first saw the blue ice, for which glaciers are famous. We also saw little blue icebergs during this part of the cruise; some with seals resting on them.

The next port of call was Juneau, Alaska's state capitol, with the magnificent Mendenhall Glacier. Our bus tour of Juneau displayed a number of points of interest including the University of Alaska local museums, restaurants, souvenir stores, and other tourist attractions. The bus system allowed stopping at points of interest, and catching the following buses on only one single fare. The most impressive thing to us on the bus tour was a stop at the edge of town, where a parking lot had a view of mighty Mendenhall in the distance. From behind I photographed Dave, admiring it. It was a pleasure, watching Dave viewing a number of the sights that he had waited so long to see. Next, we took a side trip to Mendenhall, a few miles out of Juneau. The weather was overcast, somewhat foggy and now started to drizzle, but the subject was so impressive that we didn't mind. We visited the little museum, which with its detailed geologic history, provided a better understanding of the glacier.

Skagway, the next stop, had one of our favorite attractions, the excursion on the White Pass and Yukon Railroad, which followed the main path of the forty-niners to the Yukon gold rush. This was about twenty miles through the White Pass, cut by the Skagway River. It was over narrow gage tracks to save weight, but also because there wasn't much room to lay rail and allowed for sharper turns. It was very steep with many magnificent vistas, some so sharply down that it was impossible to see the bottom on the train side. The scenic wonders, viewed out the windows of the vintage rail cars included glaciers, waterfalls, tunnels and trestle bridges. We had the cameras out snapping pictures almost constantly. When we got back to Skagway there was still time to enjoy a dramatic retelling of the death of Soapy Smith. During this drama I started feeling ill but I didn't tell Dave for fear of spoiling his vacation.

Prince Rupert, Canada was our last stop before cruising back to Seattle. Another small boat trip provided the best whale watching of the entire trip. We saw a humpback whale and her calf, and in another area several killer whales, known as orcas, feeding. By now, I just barely managed to enjoy the views because of feeling hot and nauseous but continuing to hide my discomfort from Dave.

It was an incredible trip that we will never forget. We saw the wonderful vistas and wildlife of Ketchikan, Juneau, and Skagway in Alaska, and Prince Rupert in Canada. Some of our favorite times were watching the humpback and killer whales and the dolphins do their things. The humpbacks came within clear view, through the binoculars provided, and put on a wonderful show. I felt like they knew we were watching and put on the show just for us.

Feeling ill from the last part of Skagway, and not saying anything to anyone, was the worst part of the trip. I especially did not tell Dave for fear that he would force me to go to the ship's doctor. He would have put me in the ship's infirmary. I waited until we got home to say that I felt like I could pass out. Dave took my temperature and found that I had a fever of almost 105 degrees. This is where it gets a little fuzzy for me. Dave spent the next day driving down the fever with aspirin and Tylenol. When he couldn't keep the high temperature down, he took me to the hospital. I protested that this wasn't necessary; because hospitals are for sick people. The hospital gave me tests for two days to find the cause of the fever. Finally, at my suggestion, they checked my urine, and found that I had contracted legionnaire's disease, which had progressed into legionella pneumonia. This kept me in the hospital a week, and required rest at home for another week. My week of vacation had become three weeks off from work. That was not the end of it; I was still quite weak and for the next week Dave drove me to and from work to ease some of the burden.

A TECHNOLOGICAL ORGANIZATION

After a few months, I went to work at a technological organization to get a job, about ten minutes from home, as a forty hour per week file clerk at a little more than my annual pay at the lab at thirty hours weekly. The inducement to accept a step down in responsibility was the interview statement that I would be responsible to reorganize the large file room to make it more efficient. The files were arranged in an overcomplicated system and were shared among ten immediate office employees beside other occasional personnel with need for them. They removed file folders for their use without indicating where, or by whom, they were taken.

With a proposed increase in efficiency in mind, I looked at the fifty or sixty file cabinets, and almost immediately, recommended the required use of 'out' cards, showing date removed, and initials of the removing person. I also suggested a simpler system with less places to look for files. My supervisor approved the 'out' cards, but delayed the reorganization of the files. Unfortunately she didn't enforce 'out' cards usage, so that looking for missing files could involve possibly a dozen different places, besides ordinary misfiling mistakes. This took an awful lot of my time, with individual searches for missing files often taking a half hour and sometimes considerably more.

Lost time searching for missing files, and difficulty adapting to the requirement of asking permission to make simple changes, in this more tightly supervised atmosphere, appears to have caused my supervisor to lose confidence in me. An example of the tighter supervision was my inserting newly added pages into a procedures manual. This required obtaining permission from my supervisor before I changed the pages even though the page additions were furnished and insertion was required by departmental directive. I couldn't even imagine that following the directive wasn't allowed without first asking permission of my supervisor. I had worked with considerable independence for the lab director, who would have thought I'd lost my mind, if I wasted his time, asking permission to place newly revised pages in a manual as directed.

Also I had only been there about two months when my brother, Johan, died. This required me to deal with his week of hospital intensive care, death, and protracted release of his body, insurance issues, and setting up an estate. With all this going on, my concentration was not completely on my work. With the mentioned work and home problems I lost the confidence of my supervisor, and we agreed that things were not working out. The main problems were that she wanted change in the office, while not enforcing even the simple change of 'out' card use, and that I was having problems with her much tighter supervision, and somewhat distracted by the problems surrounding Johan's death.

JOHAN'S DEATH
AND BURIAL

In February, I received a phone call from Phil, my brother, in California, that Johan was in the intensive care unit of a hospital in Washington, D. C. With the estrangement between us, Johan and I didn't have one another's addresses and with Johan's significant other having only Phil's phone number, she was unable to contact me. I rushed from work with Dave to the hospital to find Johan in a coma. His head was bloated with tubes draining fluid from it and other tubes pumping blood and intravenous medications to other parts of his body in a desperate attempt to keep him alive. It was shocking to see my vigorous forty five year old brother in that condition. The nurse told me that Johan had received massive damage to the back of his head and his brain. The tubes were to relieve the trauma caused blood pressure in his brain, which had been ten times normal and had virtually destroyed his brain function. The damage was so severe from the pressure alone that he would surely die. This was later confirmed in more detail, by the doctor. Phil flew in from California the next day. We went back to the hospital that night, and he was as shocked as I. Johan was in intensive care a week before he died in March.

It was awful. His lady friend considered him her common law husband and allowed unrestricted visits and flow of information concerning Johan's condition. A number of their friends poured through the intensive care unit, which Phil and I believed gave us insufficient privacy. Johan's promiscuous lifestyle made this time rather hectic, with his current partner and at least two other apparent loves in attendance. One of these was from a past affair. The other sweet young thing told me that Johan and she were to have been married within a week. This was in addition to his lady landlord who believed herself to be his common-law wife. There was so much tension between the possible bride to be and the current partner, and especially one of the partner's friends that I had to have the friend removed from the intensive care unit by hospital security.

We also received word that another paramour, who he had been visiting in Australia a month or so earlier, was pregnant with his child. Other admiring women, across the country, contacted us as his death became known. His local friends were still in and out of his room, which limited opportunity for Phil's and my private visiting. It seemed to me like a circus. We decided to control visitation and flow of information to provide us a little more privacy. Phil and I visited Johan every night, but the original diagnosis had been correct; he was going to die. The hospital was doing everything they could to save him, but his brain function fell to the level of virtual nonexistence, at which point, he was legally brain dead with no hope of recovery. Then they were able, legally, to ask us if we wanted heavy duty life support removed. Recognizing the hopelessness of his recovery, we approved its removal and Johan's body died.

Comments made by Johan's significant other, of a violent argument in their home between the boyfriend of Johan's about possibly new wife to be and Johan caused the Washington, D. C. Police to assume that there was a possibility his death might be a murder, and his body was not released for burial until cause of death was determined by the Medical Examiner. Over three weeks later, the Examiner determined that damage to Johan's brain was not limited to the cell damage in the immediate area, which produced the terrible pressure increase, but also included separation of two major parts of the brain. The determination was death, due to damage from a massive epileptic seizure, possibly caused by the presence of a sexually performance enhancing drug [not indicated for an epileptic] that was found in his system.

We were fortunate that Johan had chosen to have insurance deducted at work, in order to have money to bury him. There were three life policies: a life policy paid by his employer, a life policy and an accidental death policy paid by him. These enabled us to pay for his funeral and burial contingent on payment after release of his insurance to his estate, which we would have to set up. The estate process was necessary, because Johan hadn't selected beneficiaries, and the insurance would only pay his estate. This takes a minimum of six months to settle in the District of Columbia. We were the only family members left, and one of us had to set up the estate. With Phil living in California, and me in the D. C. area, I was the logical person. So it fell to me to set up and manage the estate.

The funeral wasn't too difficult, since a friend recommended a fine little funeral home, willing to accept payment after the estate was settled. Our church was very helpful, actually not requesting any payment for use of their building and staff to plan and perform the service, even including printing the programs and providing live music.

The cemetery was another matter. We contacted a large commercial cemetery and explained that money wouldn't be available until after the estate was settled. They said that they would be able to work out arrangements with us. But three days before the funeral was to take place, they told us that we would have to pay the entire cost up front. I told them that we would have to get back to them, and began looking for another cemetery. The search disclosed a small local cemetery maintained by volunteers. Their manager accepted contingency, and provided a nice little plot, under a tree as I wished, at about half the price the other cemetery wanted. Best of all, the grave was dug immediately, so that there to be no delay, which would have been a huge problem, since newspaper announcements had already been made and funeral programs printed. Naturally, we cancelled arrangements with the commercial cemetery. When we told our funeral director of this development, he said that he had heard of this problem before with the commercial cemetery and that he had good experiences with the cemetery, I had chosen. Purchase of the grave marker was delayed until after the settlement.

Johan's death was especially difficult. Although I loved him we were estranged by his conman, thieving, promiscuous ways. Our parents should have disciplined him when he started stealing from us. It might have put an end to much of the destructive behavior that I kept hearing about while I had contact with him. People he was living with, phoned me in hopes that I could retrieve money or valuables, he had stolen from them. All that I could do was recommend that they file charges with the police. He wasn't welcome in my home, because I didn't want to have deal with his stealing and promiscuousness any further. He apparently didn't want to hear my disapproval, because when I tried to contact him via the internet, he didn't respond.

The week that Phil spent with us during Johan's last days was the beginning of a renewed closeness between us that had been lost over the years because of his problems with drugs. His wife had divorced him because of his drug use and his related irresponsible behavior, which she believed to be dangerous for their infant. After the divorce he disappeared from their lives, failing to respond to attempts at contact. Over the years, I developed a love for his daughter, Laura and found his apparent desertion difficult to forgive.

This time together gave us the chance to talk. We exchanged information about why we behaved the way we did, how we had changed, and, hopefully, grown. We expressed the desire to continue to grow the relationship. Our discussions resulted in healing of some past hurts; and enlightened us as we discovered things that we didn't know about our lives. For example, Phil didn't remember that when he was two or three years old, Dad was going to spank him for something, for which he was too young, to be punished severely. As the nine year old sister, I told Dad that Phil was too young, and to spank me instead. Dad did. This, along with other things helped Phil understand how much I care about him.

I learned from Phil that after the divorce, he took a good look at himself, and decided to put his life back together. He believed that he was in no condition to be a good parent and that it was better to be no parent, than one that, based on past experience, might be a huge disappointment to his wife and daughter. He said it was because of this that he relinquished parental rights; and allowed his daughter to be adopted by his former wife's new husband.

Also he reported that in his struggle to change, he became more of a believing Christian. After overcoming his drug addiction, he had remarried. Today, instead of being supported by his wife, he and his new wife have three children, which he fully supports, while she is solely a mother, instead of a mother/wage earner. Understanding these things has helped me forgive him for the mistakes of the past, and what I had considered a desertion of his family. This made us closer than we had been at any time since Phil was an early teenager. We communicate by phone/internet to check on personal and family developments. God truly works in mysterious ways.

DONATING JOHAN'S ORGANS

When we were teenagers, my brothers and I agreed that, if we were to die, we wanted our organs donated for others' use. Phil and I decided to act on this with Johan's body. While he was in intensive care, we were informed that, with the massive trauma to his brain, he would surely die. So when we were asked by The Washington Regional Transplant Consortium if we were interested in donating his organs we immediately agreed. The Consortium, since renamed The Washington Regional Transplant Community, arranged for donation of his organs. This procedure allows some body parts to be used by persons needing them and others for medical research. The selected parts were taken immediately after the death of his body, so that they would be fresh, enough to be useful. There was an open casket funeral since removal of the parts was handled in a way not disturbing to his appearance in the casket. At the time we didn't realize the full significance of organ donation. Kidneys, for example, are in great demand with long waiting lists for people needing them. For the more serious cases it is a case of life or death.

When Johan's significant other discovered that we intended to donate parts of Johan's body, she contacted a friend's friend who needed a kidney. She suggested to her, and to us that we might consider privately donating one of his kidneys to her. This young professional woman, whom we will call Angel, had been waiting for a kidney for a long time, and was considered to be in the last few weeks of her life if she didn't receive a successful transplant quickly. Angel mailed us personal information: her medical condition, and work, and family situations. This revealed that she was a responsible midlevel government employee and single mother, with very limited life expectancy, without a transplant. We decided that we would like to help; and designated Angel to receive one of Johan's kidneys. This had the added possibility, of substituting for the sister that I had wanted, especially after the death of my infant sister, so many years ago.

Sometime after the transplant procedure, when there was a chance that significant healing had taken place, we left word through The Washington Regional Transplant Community, (the new name), that we would like to know how Angel was doing, and if she was interested in meeting us. She responded that she was much better, hoped to return to work soon, and wanted to meet us. After a few months at work, Angel had a business trip that brought her within an hour's ride of our home. We invited her to visit on that weekend, and had a merry time at home, talking extensively, introducing her to our favorite card game and taking her to the large church that we attended.

Angel thoroughly enjoyed the service, and since we had developed a mutual interest in encouraging human organ transplantation, we pointed out that they might be interested in a presentation. If they were, we decided that she might be able tell the church how much a new kidney meant to her on her next scheduled visit to the area. After checking with the pastor, the presentation was scheduled. The Washington Regional Transplant Community provided promotional brochures, and the presentation was held as we planned. She told her story to two morning services at church, to audiences totaling roughly five thousand people.

During her visits, we found strong mutual interests and enjoyed our time together. We were invited to visit, when it could be arranged with her, in San Francisco, and her parents at their home a little way down the coast.

SETTLING JOHAN'S
ESTATE

Setting up an estate is a complicated process and I wanted to find a capable attorney in estate settlement. Before taking Mom across country, I had worked for a settlement attorney who had long since retired, but could refer me. I told him my problem and he mentioned a reputable law firm. They told us that Phil and I would have to decide on an executor, either one of us or a third party; and that with executor charges; it might as well be one of us. With Phil living in California and my living in the Washington, DC metro area, I was the obvious choice. We signed several forms at the attorney's office to set it up. In the District of Columbia an estate must remain open for six months in order to pay all of the final estate bills. Each month the law firm sent me the bills. I wrote the checks and mailed them. There was a substantial amount at the end. Phil and I split the proceeds of the estate right down the middle, except for my modest executor fees established by law. It saddens me that, for a number of years, I had very little relationship with my brothers. They had lived too far away and had copied many of Dad's and Johan's bad habits. Growing up in a dysfunctional family may have had a lot to do with it. I don't think they knew how much I loved them; and wish things could have been different. For parts of this that are my fault I am truly sorry.

Since Johan's and Mike's deaths, I think Phil and I have at times been closer than we were before. The saying, "death can either tear you apart or bring you closer," seems to be true.

GETTING LIGHT BOXES

My psoriasis was not responding enough to satisfy my fine dermatologist. She prescribed the use of her light box every other day. Light boxes are cabinets containing a number of specialized tube lamps of extremely bright light. They are like tanning devices but much more powerful and brighter, requiring both a doctor's prescription and very gradual increase in time of exposure. Even though she reduced the price to ten dollars a visit I found this a drain on our budget and decided to see if there was some way to obtain a light box. A search of the internet produced an advertisement for a used full body box. It was owned by a man in New Hampshire, who had just retired and was moving to Florida. He expected to spend a lot of time in the sun fishing, golf, etc. Release from the tension of work, combined with all that sunshine seemed to him to overcome the need for a light box. His sale price was forty seven hundred dollars, reasonable for a nearly new professional box. Unfortunately, I couldn't afford anything near that amount. So I e mailed a no thank you. He reduced the price to thirty seven hundred. I still couldn't afford it but accepted his final offer of twenty five hundred dollars.

Dave and I got some rope, bungee cords and blankets and headed to New Hampshire. This was to be a jolly trip and getting there was, except for our making a wrong turn in northern New Jersey and having to make a twenty or thirty mile correction in the crazy traffic of the metropolitan New York City area. We arrived at our destination in the early afternoon and, after meeting this charming couple, inspected the equipment with its paper work and related two pairs of very dark glasses to protect our eyes from the extreme brilliance of the light. Everything was in excellent condition with the original certificate of official inspection that was fully adequate because the box was so new. We flattened the back seat of the car and with the help of the seller took the box out to load in our car. This was done with great care because each of the ten light tubes in the box cost over a hundred dollars and if one was damaged all would have to be replaced.

We headed for home with Dave hoping to arrive that night. We took a different route in order to avoid the crazy driving that we met on the way up. Dave is very project oriented and was intent on being home in Maryland that night. It started to rain lightly shortly after leaving New Hampshire, but Dave was still trying get home that night. He hoped to save us the cost of a motel and extra meals on the road. We soon found ourselves on an empty high speed highway but eighty miles an hour in the dark in the rain is ridiculous. Fortunately a state police officer interrupted this craziness and blessed us with a ticket after pointing out that he was trying to save our lives. We stopped for the night at the first motel. The next morning, despite the rain, the box was undamaged and we headed home in a more leisurely fashion.

Over time I found that the full body box we had purchased, while excellent for most of my body, was not adequate for my hands and feet. It was especially poor for the psoriasis on my feet which needed a specialized box designed for that purpose. The research started again. This time there was nothing used available that seemed appropriate. I looked for an established manufacturer and found the nearest one, with a competitively low price, in Ohio. Checking with them reminded me that I had to have a prescription from my dermatologist the same as with the full body box, purchased earlier. We headed for Ohio and found the trip much more pleasant because of the natural beauty and the consideration of the drivers on the road. There was none of the extreme rushing and aggressive driving that we had encountered in the larger New York City metropolitan area. The people at the factory were very helpful, pointing out a good inexpensive restaurant and an inexpensive motel for the night. The next day they helped us load the car and we headed home. We came home with a very pleasant opinion of people and drivers in Ohio, who seemed very considerate.

As time went by I found using the heavy hand and foot light box uncomfortable because if on the floor for feet it is uncomfortable for hands. If on a table for hands it is uncomfortable for feet. This is especially true after using the box for a while and building the time of individual exposure from a few seconds to fifteen to twenty minutes or more. I phoned the manufacturer to see if they had a solution to this problem. Their answer was to buy another box. At twenty five hundred dollars this didn't appeal. Dave thought about the problem and considered several possible design solutions. Finally he decided that a tilt table system seemed to be simplest. He has most of the basic equipment but hasn't implemented it yet because he doesn't have an engineering background and without knowledge of strength of materials is afraid that I could get hurt if the table broke from excessive design pressures in the use of the table. He is still looking for assistance with that problem.

Using light boxes requires great care. It is not difficult to be burned severely which is why it is done with a prescription under the care of a physician. Early in my use of the full body box I burned myself severely. I accidentally entered the time of usage as ten minutes instead of a minute. This produced second degree burns over my entire body except for my head which had been covered. At first I had to keep all the window blinds closed because the pain was so great that the touch of clothing was intolerable. After a few days my skin was peeling off in sheets. It took months before I could get back into the light box. The purpose of the light box is to help control my psoriasis and it is helpful when I use it properly. There have been times I have just gotten so tired of it and let it go. When that happens, I break out worse and then I have to start over in my light treatments with a very few seconds and gradually build the time back up. Treatments have to be done every other day. Psoriasis is not a contagious disease but it is chronic and incurable although sometimes it will go into remission for a while. Winter weather is very dry and hard on the skin and my skin tends to break and crack in the winter time. Unfortunately, stress also makes it worse and my worrying doesn't help. I am only able to use special skin products like Dove soap and shampoo,

Psoriasis is a difficult skin disorder to live with. It itches me like crazy when it breaks out. Use of cold packs helps with the itching and I am forever using ointments, creams, light boxes, etc. On occasion use of plastic gloves helps to heal my hands. Winter is the worst time for me. I constantly wash my hands which also aggravates psoriasis. It is better than it has been in a long time. Originally, I was misdiagnosed with eczema instead of psoriasis by my group health management organization. When I cancelled my policy and started with another insurance company I started seeing doctors that were PPO (no referral needed for an appointment). I found this wonderful dermatologist who has seen me through some very hard times. She is both my dermatologist and my friend. I am very grateful to her and her staff. I still see her occasionally for psoriasis and other skin ailments as they pop up even though we have moved up to Pennsylvania.

CHURCH COUNSELING

After Johan died Dave and I applied for and received counseling from our church. This was mostly Dave's idea He believed that he was taking the role of teacher too often. It is role that he finds comfortable, but he thought it was interfering with our relationship as married partners. Also, with my negative outlook on life, I was having difficulty handling the stresses in a very difficult work adjustment at my new job with the technological organization and the problems accompanying Johan's death. They finally resulted in loss of that job. Dave wanted help in modifying his behavior and for me to have help with my stresses. There was no charge for the counseling, but we tried to give the church as much as we were able. We also appreciated the wonderful teaching, fellowship and kindnesses that they had provided over the years. When we were married by the pastor of the church, they gave us a small cash wedding present and charged us nothing for the costs of the ceremony. Also, they had been very generous in charging us nothing to provide funeral services for Johan's funeral. The counselor decided that my stresses were the most pressing issue and decided to try and work with them first. We went to the counseling for awhile after Johan's death.

Talking about problems and our relationship (the little bit that we dealt with that) helped some. But we never really finished the counseling because of new job type pressures and my not really wanting to deal with my problems and stresses at that time. I just wanted to forget everything. The counseling actually added to my stress because of my not being willing to deal just then. This added stressful activity did not help in trying to learn a new job. I was a mess. Why? Why me? Why wouldn't Phil take responsibility for the estate? I asked him and he said, "Oh, yeah, but I live in California and it would make more sense if you handled it." I told him, I did not want to handle it and asked couldn't he manage to take care of it?

I don't think Phil realized how devastating it was for me. I loved Johan but I could never get my brother back since he had decided to live in the fast lane. I couldn't keep up with him and didn't want to, but would have liked a reasonable relationship with him. Sometimes I think Phil had a difficult time keeping up with him, too. I never thought anything as devastating as his early death and the manner of it would have happened. It is a blessing that Mom was not around to see it. Mike's and Johan's deaths and Johan's life style and behaviors would have broken her heart. She loved all of us so very much, and raised us to be honorable and responsible.

HOSPITALIZED

Johan's difficult death, the trouble of getting him buried, problems setting up the estate, and worries about my new job were wearing on me heavily. The job at the technical organization hadn't been successful. The employer was not happy and neither was I. I had lost my job. Things finally got to be too much. As I had done in the past, in slicing my wrist with a knife, while homeless, and jumping out the third floor window to escape what appeared to me to be an impossible situation, I tried to escape. I told Dave that I was going to take an overdose of sleeping pills. I did, but not enough to kill me. Then I ran out of the house with car keys and drove around the area, to have time to think things over. While this was going on, Dave, not knowing what to expect, and not wanting me to die, called the police to find me, calm me down and get me back home. I phoned Dave from the car. He asked me to come home, so that we could talk and decide what to do. I thought, maybe we could work this out. When I drove into our parking lot, the police, who had been looking all over, were waiting for me.

Dave wanted them to let it go at that, but they wouldn't. They insisted on taking me to a local hospital where I was installed in the psych ward. After a few days I was transferred to an adjacent mental facility, where they kept me for a week, until they decided it was safe to discharge me. But they insisted on a short period of counseling. I attended counseling sessions individually and with Dave for a few times before we let it lapse and that was the end of it.

PHOTOGRAPHY

By the end of the of the estate settlement in November, my favorite thirty five millimeter film camera that we had purchased earlier, and used heavily on our trips, had broken. I had loved taking photographs from the time that my parents bought me the Polaroid Land Camera, when I was a teenager. The estate settlement enabled me to indulge myself a little. So Dave and I decided to look at buying a new digital model. They are a huge technological improvement, because they provide instant pictures, without the delay of film processing, or the cost of film. There is no film and the images, stored electronically in the camera on an electronic chip, are erasable at the minimal cost of the very slight drain on the battery. Furthermore, digital image quality is improving, and is very nearly as good as, or equal to what can be obtained from everything, except the most specialized and expensive film and development. We went to a camera store and purchased a Canon Power Shot A650 IS. It is very sensitive for a point and shoot camera with its 12.1 mega pixel sensor. Its 6X optical zoom lens also provides a reasonable amount of flexibility. This was not the digital single lens reflex camera (DSLR) that I had been thinking about. But it was much less expensive, yet sensitive and versatile enough, to allow me to take pictures that could be enlarged to poster size without appreciable loss of image quality. With its less complicated menu, it helped me learn to use some of the functions available on single lens reflex cameras. I was very excited about my new toy, and started shooting pictures around the neighborhood. It began to feel comfortable to use, and I soon learned most of the menu functions. It was ideal as a learning camera, complex enough for considerable variety and sensitive enough for poster pictures because of the qualities of the sensor and lens. The menu eased my learning how to use it and the zoom increased the variety of its image capturing capability.

Dave and I had been looking for an activity that we could mutually enjoy. He also began to shoot a few pictures occasionally. This appeared to be a hobby that we could do together. Dave was very rusty at picture taking and I believed that I needed help in photography. So we took a course in photography together at a local college, enrolling in the same course, running three months. The course was taught by a charismatic teacher, a highly successful local photographer. He was very inspirational in his approach to teaching, allowing considerable freedom to class members in how to carry out assignments. He had a mantra of "shoot, shoot, shoot." As if this wasn't enough incentive, the class had a policy, of providing loaner digital single lens reflex (DSLR) cameras, for a week at a time, on alternate weeks. Between the two of us, we could select alternate weeks, and if there wasn't too much student demand, have at least one school DSLR between us for almost the entire course. It worked out very well; we had a one of several Nikon D40s nearly the whole time. With the practice I already had shooting my Canon Power Shot; I found the move to the Nikon D40 relatively easy. Dave found it a little bit more difficult, because he had much less practice with the Power Shot.

The class was for three hours twice a week in addition to required extensive shooting of many examples of nine or ten specific types of photographs. It required attendance at well illustrated lectures, study of course materials, and study of a famous photographer with a 250 word report on his/her work. Dave and I both chose Ansel Adams, the great creator of black and white nature pictures; innovator in film development, teacher, and powerhouse in American photography. We worked completely independently on our reports and were graded well on them. It also required lab work outside and in taking portraits in the college studios. The final test was the winnowing of our pictures in each of the picture types to a single selection with each of us printing his/her pictures on college equipment and producing final images on the listed specific types of subjects. These we matted, and mounted for portfolios, which were the final test. The portfolios were judged by the Head of the Photographic Department, and our professor. We were not the best in the class which had some other students with much more photographic experience and their own high quality equipment. But we both came out with grades of B and were delighted to have done that well with so little knowledge entering the class. We found it interesting that our main interests were both in photographing natural beauty in landscapes although with very different approaches. My interest was in framing the picture in its natural background, to increase the emotional impact, which conflicted with the objective of basic training in a first course in photography. Dave's interest was in picturing very simple, but still esthetically interesting objects either with very simple backgrounds or in their natural settings. We both enjoyed the course, but I was no longer satisfied with the canon, and, instead, wanted a much more versatile professional quality DSLR.

CONTRACTING AT ANOTHER SCIENTIFIC ORGANIZATION

Next I obtained work for a contractor with another scientific organization at more pay as administrative assistant to the director of one of the labs. He was new, hired six months earlier. My supervisor, the lab manager, was hired two weeks before me. His work for the same organization with the contractor, so impressed them that they bought his release from the contract, to promote him to more responsibility as a staff employee. Most of his previous work had been similar to mine as travel planner/ timekeeper. We got off to a good cooperative start, volunteering some weekend work together, relocating our office. For a while cooperation was the norm. He seemed to enjoy my organization of my work station, and ideas such as using my new camera to create a poster, of the laboratory staff with the director in the middle of it.

However, he soon seemed rattled by the change in status, unsure of some of the duties that I already knew, and very uncomfortable with being a supervisor, which he said he didn't want to be. Because he had worked there, I asked him questions about procedures, which might be particular to the way they operated. This presented problems, because he claimed to be too busy to answer my questions. Never-the-less he demanded that I address all of my questions to him. After a lack of timely necessary answers, I told him that I had to have prompt answers in order to do my work, and that my training was part of his responsibility. He disagreed. When his failures to respond interfered with the ability to do my job, I told him that I had to obtain answers about work wherever they could be found. This made our relationship very difficult, because he resented my looking elsewhere, when his answers were not forthcoming.

I told my contracting work supervisor about the trouble I was having with the lab manager. He was insisting that I wasn't carrying enough of the workload. By refusing to train me or answer my questions in a timely manner he interfered with my ability to do my job. The contracting work supervisor had been his contracting supervisor, and said that he would talk with him, but it did no good. So, when after several weeks, I spoke to him again, he recommended that I prepare a spread sheet. This was to show what, and when work was received, performed, and passed on. I did, and found that I appeared to be doing almost all of the work including work for which I had not been trained. When this came to the attention of management, they asked me, why I was doing almost all the work including that for which they had trained him. I said he had told me to do the work. This meant that I had to seek help because I hadn't been trained. By this time, the lab manager had become more and more agitated, telling me that he had sent hateful memos to people in management, and I overheard him throw a violent verbal tantrum in the lab director's office.

Shortly after this he was discharged, and they said he told them I wasn't doing my share of the work. Believing this, they had decided to let both of us go. They said they had to let us go in order to solve the problem of lack of production, and that it wasn't until after they saw the spread sheet, that they discovered I was doing practically all of the work. When they found out that I was doing both his work and mine, they had already obligated his job to another experienced employee and eliminated mine. They said that they were sorry, because I had been doing a good job, but it was too late to do anything about the change. They gave me some nice reference letters and that was that. I worked for them for about 5 months as a contractor. It was disappointing that the job lasted so short a time. I really enjoyed it and the people there, but it just didn't work out.

ANOTHER TECHNICAL
ORGANIZATION

In September of 2008 I received an unofficial phone call from a technical organization that I had been selected for a job that would pay me more than I had earned before. They said it might be soon pending a clearance which could take up to six months. Dave and I were excited, finally to have found familiar work. Since I had become very competent in these particular duties over the course of several years, this assignment seemed like a piece of cake. We immediately bought the Nikon D300 camera that I had been planning for, when permanently employed. I had wanted it since taking the camera course and we considered ourselves fortunate to be able to find a good used Nikon 2.8 medium zoom lens at the store at the same time. We decided to get many of the basic needs and bought a quality light weight tripod, a shoe mount flash attachment, filters, extra batteries and memory cards. What fun! But it was awfully expensive, the most, that we had spent, except for a house or car. Dave knew that I really enjoy photography and the DSLR was a dream come true a considerable step up from the DSLR we borrowed in the camera course. It was a true professional model camera with similar quality related equipment.

We considered that, with scenic travel, one of our major passions, we could go on trips with our new photographic equipment and capture great landscape pictures! Also, some things had happened that encouraged thoughts, that my passion for photography had the possibility of being profitable. My dentist admired my picture of the huge sculpture, located on the lawn outside of his office and asked us to print one in eight and one half by eleven size to display on the office wall. It turned out that his partner nixed this idea, but it was very encouraging. One of his employees made patchwork quilts which she hoped to make into a profitable sideline. She offered to pay me to make photos of her work for advertising purposes. Also, when I was working at the previous job there was considerable interest in my making poster size photos of our group to hang in the office area.

This new job proved to be very disappointing. The training on specialized software and procedures was very limited and the little which was informally provided was inadequate. I had applied for a position near my home but management planned to have me work in Washington, D.C. I didn't want to work in Washington because the local job allowed me to be closer to home. If Dave needed me for a return of his severe vertigo attacks, I would be only twenty minutes from home locally versus an hour or more in Washington. After a day of being forced by management to work in Washington, the union was able to have me assigned near home. I was grateful that this job was in a union.

Never-the-less it was disappointing, since I was continually asked to ignore proper rules and regulations. The original job announcement and the job description both indicated the job was to be responsible for proper use of these rules and regulations. I had signed documents promising to uphold them. It seemed that it was going to be great but my experience there shows how wrong you can be. Instead I had to struggle with management, mostly in the person of my supervisor to enforce proper rules and regulations. Five months later I was told I would be receiving my progress review which was my supervisor's lie. When he came to our campus, supposedly to give me a performance review he presented me with a letter of termination, quite different from a progress review. As permitted by the union agreement, I had told him that I wanted a union representative present because of a grievance I had filed against him because of the rule and regulation problems. He scheduled the alleged progress review when the union representative was out of town in order to deny me my rights under the agreement. I was asked to leave the building and did but still pursued the already filed grievance. I believe this termination was due to my attempts to comply with rules and regulations and the grievance filed against him and was an act of reprisal.

Shortly thereafter I attended a meeting with Human Resources people and my union representative. He did most of the talking regarding my grievance; however, I found his protection of my union rights very poor! He failed to deal with the issues of the grievance and seemed to agree that I be terminated which I believe to be wrongful. Dave and I had visited the union representative at his beloved recently purchased obviously unprofitable enterprise and had real questions about where the money for the purchase and to keep it afloat was coming from. The fact that he stepped down from his union position after failing to keep me quiet made us suspicious of what was going on. This combined with the purposeful ignoring of the regulations along with improprieties in other aspects of the work made us more suspicious. The constant turnover of personnel and improper delegation of important responsibilities to new untrained personnel after trained personnel had given adverse responses to management requests for approval of certain improper transactions produced a suspicion of the likelihood of corruption being hidden in purposeful confusion in relatively minor misdeeds of those forced into or complicit in the minor misdeeds in proper office procedures.

I felt disgusted with the organization. Next was a period of waiting on higher management to see what would happen. It would have been nice if they could have managed to be fair and put me in a different department. I was getting a very uncomfortable and uneasy feeling about this whole thing.

It was a real disappointment that my manager insisted people to do things that were wrong, appalling!! In order to do my job, I needed a supervisor that would 1) honor rules and regulations, 2) not pressure me for trying to obey them and 3) provide adequate training. These issues kept going on and on as I appealed them through various appeal processes. The end result was that I was fired. I should note that a number of fellow employees told me that they admired my courage and integrity.

SAN FRANCISCO
AND SAN JOSE

While waiting for the federal agency to complete its clearance procedure we had been invited to visit Angel (the recipient of one of Johan's kidneys) and her family in California and decided to see if a visit around either Thanksgiving or Christmas could work. We were fortunate to find a reduced airfare promotion. Between the date constraints of the reduced fare and the problem of dates of Angel's preplanned trip to Asia, a week in November worked very nicely.

So Dave and I flew to San Francisco, California to meet Angel, her son, her parents and the rest of the family. It worked spectacularly; we couldn't have planned it better. Before Dave and I left, my brother, Phil told us that he would not be able to meet with us in San Francisco. But he and Angel had planned a surprise for us. It was a party for me and is one time Phil really kept a surprise. I could usually find out more information from him than either Johan or Mike.

It was a thoroughly enjoyable trip. Phil, Dave, and I rode street cars down to Fisherman's Wharf where we walked around and had lunch. Although we didn't ride on cable cars as we had planned, we took photos of ourselves with them. I have never seen so many stores on pier after pier in the ocean as at and around Fisherman's Wharf. It was a great tourist trap with a good part of the attraction the large seals splashing in the water and on rafts nearby. Dave and I used the new Nikon D300 Camera that we had bought earlier in November. It was great planning. We had a couple of memory sticks with one holding over 400 pictures. It was hard to believe something so small could hold so much. One thing you can say for San Francisco, it is very hilly. We did plenty of walking which was great for us. I think Angel was afraid that both of us would pass out because of not being in great shape. This may be why she paid for and booked us into a pleasant motel on a main street with trolley travel, rather than have us climb the hills of her neighborhood and the many steep steps to her home.

Our first night there it made us spectators to a noisy protest of proposition 8, a new California law which defined marriage as being between a man and a woman, opposed by the gay community. The protest passed right below our windows. The law, at that time, had the effect of stopping further same sex marriages which had been approved by a judge in Northern California. It caused enormous resentment and a number of protests in the gay communities throughout California. I roused Dave, so we could witness the parade of protesters in front of our window, which lasted at least half an hour.

Angel was a wonderful hostess. Despite working, she provided an excellent dinner at her beautiful home one night. Another it was dinner at a fine Spanish restaurant. A third day she took us across San Francisco to Oakland for a delicious lunch and further down the coast to meet her parents and family. They fed us that night at a large family dinner. The food was great, the family magnificent, and the children perfectly charming. Part of the fun was playing Black Outs, our favorite card game with her family. We had taught Angel this when she visited our home and she had taught her family. It. was a great evening. Finally she showed us the golden gate bridge and Alcatraz. What a delightful trip!

MORE VISITS TO LAURA

Dave and I went to Laura's huge high school graduation. At the outdoor stadium's stage she received her diploma and played in the school's marching band ceremonies. Laura graduated third in her large class with high honors and scholarships, jump starting University of Georgia classes with advanced placement courses. She is earning a Bachelor degree in Recreation and Leisure Studies for a missionary career in camp work in Africa. One class took her to Russia to a Christian camp in one of her courses. Yorba and Swahili, her language studies are expected to help equip her in parts of East and West Africa. After graduation, she is engaged to be married to her high school sweetheart, a fine young military man.

Returning to the house at night after graduation ceremonies Dave and I encountered a Georgia State police officer. Guided by our navigation system, Dave was driving through an unlit torn up work area with orange pylons and barrels. The state police officer was ahead of us driving toward us on the same road. With the road torn up and in the dark, Dave got into the oncoming lane and both he and the officer had to make last minute corrections in order to avoid a collision. Both stopped and Dave got out of the car saying, "I'm glad to see you." The officer said," Well, I'm not glad to see you." He checked to see if Dave had been drinking. He hadn't and explained that he had become confused in the dark in unfamiliar territory and felt lost. Then the officer asked if I drove. When I said, "Yes," he asked how long we would be in Georgia. After hearing that it would only be a day or so he told me to drive and, after giving directions, sent us on our way. We assumed that he was glad to have us out of Georgia soon. No ticket. Whew!!

On Thanksgiving, Dave and I made a four day trip to Georgia to celebrate and help with the local annual Ronald McDonald House charity dinner. Virginia and Dan again allowed us to stay at their home. Virginia told us they usually help with final preparation and serving of the ample meal. This one had turkey, ham, stuffing, gravy, vegetables, mashed potatoes, yams with marshmallows homemade pies, whipped cream and cookies, ice cream, coffee, sodas, and other trimmings I've forgotten. This massive dinner with its group of regular volunteers was accomplished very smoothly and I met a lot of nice people, many from homeless shelters. I had been unaware of this part of Ronald McDonald operations and learned something that day about how I could help people. The drive to Georgia plus this effort left us tired upon returning to Laura's home, "full as a tick" from this great meal and glad to have helped in a charity this worthwhile.

I have been blessed to be involved in the lives of Laura and her half brother, Pat, who is expecting to follow his sister's educational success if not her path of endeavor. They are apples of my eye and I enjoy my relationships with each of them.

On Sunday we went to Church with Laura and her beau. Dave told the minister afterward that we enjoyed the service. The next day he met with Dave revealing that he wanted to start a ministry. He discovered the minister was new there. They exchanged suggestions about starting and strengthening ministries. Dave enjoyed the minister's suggestions and his apparent appreciation of Dave's suggestions before they went their separate ways, possibly to reconnect later.

DILLSBURG,
PENNSYLVANIA

After three years of looking for administrative work and with unemployment compensation exhausted, the high costs of living in Montgomery County, Maryland were eating heavily into our savings. With my twenty or so medical problems, I had applied for Social Security Disability benefits. After two years of waiting, my disability application was denied; so I hired a lawyer to reapply. Dave and I decided to move to a less expensive area. Reduction of our living costs was getting urgent, so we seriously considered his daughter Deb's suggestion of mobile homes in the Gettysburg area. It would be good to be near Deb, who is a dear friend and within driving distance of our doctors, who were very good to us. Also living expenses would be lower. We engaged Pam, an excellent real estate sales woman, who drove us crazy ridding ourselves of twenty years clutter to make our home saleable. She recommended a number of expensive changes and dressed the house. This made it look gorgeous and enabled its sale in three days in a very difficult real estate market at the going rate on comparable housing in our neighborhood.

Surfing the net to find mobile home information led me to a realtor for mobile homes. She took us to see six or seven homes in several mobile home communities in the Gettysburg/Harrisburg area. We were especially impressed with two double wide homes in attractive communities, one in New Oxford and one in Dillsburg. We selected the one in Dillsburg. It had a number of advantages. It was the most attractive site in the community, a beautiful twenty foot blue spruce tree in the side yard, a lovely deck and fine flower garden in the front. The back yard is larger than the one we moved from with a larger shed and Dave planted a vegetable garden there. The home, clearly the premier location in the community, has a marvelous view from the large bay window in the kitchen looking down the hill to trees backed by low mountain ridges and, weather permitting, beautiful clouds in an exquisitely blue sky. Beside all of the above it was less expensive than the other double wide which was somewhat newer and also gorgeous.

Dillsburg, Pennsylvania is in a beautiful rural area with low mountains and rolling hills. It has lovely vistas of farms with barns, tall silos and long spreads of corn and other crops. It also has plenty of cows, a few horses and sheep with a sprinkling of more exotic creatures such as lamas and guinea hens. I don't recall living in the country earlier but I enjoy residing in such a visually beautiful area. The people here are generally very kind and helpful compared with the more formal and suspicious urban style of life in large metropolitan areas.

It has been a really exciting time for us! In November we moved into our mobile home. It is fully paid for, free and clear . . . no mortgage!! It had been repossessed by the bank and the previous owner had taken the central air conditioning unit, kitchen stove, refrigerator/freezer, washer, and dryer so these items were bought in October/November. In the following spring we made some minor roof repairs and had a new central air conditioning unit installed. It has been not only exciting but expensive as well.

Also our move to Dillsburg gradually has had the effect of deepening our religious experiences and commitments. Soon after we arrived we attended a Sunday service at the closest protestant church. It had a scripted liturgical style similar to the Catholic Church of my youth which was discouraging of my genuine personal participation. Though this style is less effective in engaging me it does not seem as stifling for everyone. Several weeks later we accepted an invitation from a neighbor to attend his large church. The teaching and style of service seemed more comfortable. But attending a discussion of a proposed church covenant caused us to be wary. This was because we believed that the proposed covenant could lead to excessive leadership control, even if it didn't start that way.

A few weeks later we stopped by another church on the way home from shopping to interview the pastor to discover what his church was like. He said there were lots of good churches in the area and he was more interested in helping us find a church where we could be comfortable and grow spiritually, than recruiting us for his. This sounded good and we decided that we would start with his. Our attendance has been regular as we have found good teaching combined with wonderful support, for both of us from church members, while Dave was in the hospital. On other occasions church members have very helpful with more simple non medical problems of equipment in our new home. Ironically this church also requires a covenant for membership but it seems less subject to abuse.

As time has gone by, I have started attending two different bible studies and find them interesting. Dave has been attending church men's breakfasts and a men's retreat and we have attended small group suppers and a church picnic. The combination of good teaching and good fellowship and real examples of The Holy Spirit in fellow church members' lives has stimulated us to apply for church membership. Reading church literature has excited me, as I have found questions about purgatory, infant baptism and role of the sacraments answered in my favor. This has been very exciting because disagreement with my entire family and church as a teenager had been very uncomfortable. This was especially so because I loved Mom so much. It has been fun to see Dave excited about being God's workmanship as this was combined with other verses about the Holy Spirit in you.

Since Dave's writing was completed I have received the benefit of a miracle. By now you know that grand mal epileptic seizures are fast in onset and that there is no time for other activity. I started to have one while I was in our car to drive a carless friend to the nearest food shopping five miles away.

When it started my first thought was I have to go inside; if the seizure happens here it will frighten my friend half to death. Then I was feeling desperate and angry. Why hadn't God permitted this to happen inside our home where it would have been less of a problem with Dave there to help me? Suddenly the cabin of the car was engulfed in a great wing of brilliant white feathers and I could no longer see my friend. Later my friend said that I said, "Okay Okay" in an angry tone of voice as I started to get out of the car. With my eyes closed against the pain of the light and feeling my way past the lamp post to and along the wood edge of the flower bed I walked along the lawn up four steps across the deck and into our home (a total of forty six steps).

Inside I held onto the doorknob to keep from falling and faintly asked Dave for help. He assisted me to the recliner where I insisted that he drive our friend to the store as I had promised. He went for his jacket but by the time he returned to the living room I was out of it, drooling and shuddering. He wouldn't leave me except for just long enough to tell our friend that we would have to shop later after I had slept for several hours to recuperate.

This turned out to be a great blessing for me for several reasons. It revealed that a new medicine I had been taking was diminishing the effectiveness of my epilepsy medicine and had to be discontinued. More importantly it overcame the doubts about whether God loves me or is able to help me which my poor relationship with Dad had made so hard to believe. He had used some of my favorite Bible verses Isaiah chapter forty verses twenty nine through thirty one to help me get into the house and to increase my belief in Him. Halleluiah!

I don't want to appear to be saying that everything is all sweetness and light in Dillsburg. My medical problems have increased with age and the extra wear and tear of the powerful drugs my body has endured in order to heal or control my roughly twenty various physical/medical malfunctions, damages and illnesses. One of the problems associated with rural life is the difficulty of getting good health care. I have just discovered that my second local primary physician is inadequate to take care of my many medical needs even to the point of not making needed referrals to specialists or following through on office details. Oh well, back to the fun of research; I'm looking for another general practitioner and a specialist to address some new troubling relatively constant nagging symptoms. But these doctors are all twenty to thirty miles away, not particularly wonderful on potentially snowy, country roads.

People are people; they haven't all become saints up here, although I can report that rural life seems to generate more kindness than urban/suburban life and that we are happier here.

POSTSCRIPT

One of the themes of this book has been the contrast between Dad's life of trying to maintain his dreams and escape from the disappointments of reality versus mine of trying to understand and embrace reality. Another is the importance of mutual loving support between husband and wife versus the damage of competition in maintaining the spousal relationship. A third theme displays, through the damage done in my life and the lives of my brothers, the importance of love and positive reinforcement in raising children. Others show the enormous strains placed on marriage by the multiple problems of severe illness, alcoholism, and frequent relocation especially when combined with the parents' failures to either understand or possibly care enough about one another's needs. No wonder we had such a dysfunctional family resulting in so much tragedy.

However, the tragedy was not unrelieved. There were fun times in the midst of it, even if a lot of them were pranks on the outside world or on Dad, which was rough on family unity. In fact, the pranks on Dad helped relieve the sorrow/horror of his drunkenness. But this same prank aggressiveness, when directed at him, discharged some of our anger at him. An example was when we took photos of him drunk with his face in his dinner plate on the table. This kind of laughter at Dad's expense was part of the warfare between my parents. It increased the separation between him and the rest of us, which his growing drunkenness and cruelty, along with Mom's competitiveness and verbal fire power had already opened up.

It seems to me now after all these years of trying to understand the causes of the destruction of our family that it was not <u>all</u> his neglect and rough treatment. Much as I love Mom and my memory of her I believe that her vicious tongue combined with his lack of self confidence and belief in God to hold on to, probably contributed to his slipping further into alcoholism and his abusive reactions. In other words, in my opinion, the only way this horrible mismatch of competitiveness, lack of male self confidence, atheism, alcoholism, huge stresses of extreme illness, the continuous moving of military life and Mom's dominance, competitiveness and verbal firepower could work was if they both had a growing understanding of God's love for them so that their dependence would have been primarily on Him rather on the fragility of human relationship. Mom loved Jesus and I'm convinced that she is in heaven but more understanding of God's great and powerful love would have been very helpful to her. I don't know if Dad is in heaven but am convinced that on that great day when everyone gets to see him clearly he'll have the opportunity that the troubles of his life may have denied him.

But life rises from the ashes, even if somewhat twisted. I have a happy and productive life although I still have problems with negative thinking and angering. Phil has grown a lot and now provides for his new wife and three children as he was not able to do for his first wife and child with the drug habit which he kicked before starting this family.

God is good. Mom didn't have to live to see Mike's suicide, Phil's difficulty with drugs which destroyed his first marriage, Johan's misspent life and unnecessary death, or my extended struggles to overcome the effects of our family dysfunctions. I have confidence in God's mercy and fairness that Mike, Johan and Dad will get a chance to clearly see Jesus as HE is in all his beauty, love, justice, mercy, and majesty. This may have been too clouded a picture for Johan and Dad to be able to recognize in their life times because of the trauma in their lives. I know that Mike loved Jesus and expect to see him in heaven. Phil has already been finding the healing of accepting God's love. He is passing it along to his family and to those he meets. I am in the midst of accepting and experiencing it also and am passing it along to the best of my ability. We both have much to offer now that we have been the recipients of so much healing and are joyful at the opportunity to share it with others. It is a delight to be God's workmanship (Ephesians 2: 8-10). Fortunately, HE isn't done with me yet; I mess up every day, but HE picks me up, washes me off with the water of his Word, and encourages me to keep on moving, knowing that HE is preparing me, and has prepared the work for me to do. What a joy life is when I have this focus. When life slips out of focus HE is with me to help me get refocused and get on with the joy. Truly HE makes his burdens light (Matt 11:30). Hallelujah!!

BIBLE VERSES THAT GOT ME THROUGH HARD TIMES

Isaiah Chapter 40:28-31 This is a favorite verse of mine and I want this book to be an encouragement to those with disabilities and those without.

Do you not know?
Have you not heard?
The Lord is the everlasting God, the Creator of the ends of the earth, He will not grow tired or weary, and his understanding no one can fathom.
He gives strength to the weary and increases the power of the weak. Even youths grow tired and weary, and young men stumble and fall; but those who hope in the Lord will renew their strength. They will soar on wings like eagles; they will run and not grow weary, they will walk and not be faint.

Isaiah Chapter 53:4-6

Surely he took up our infirmities and carried our sorrows, yet we considered him stricken by God, smitten by him, and afflicted.

But he was pierced for our transgressions, he was crushed for our inequities; the punishment that brought us peace was upon him, and by his wounds we are healed.

We all, like sheep have gone astray, each of us has turned to his own way; and the Lord has laid on him the iniquity of us all.

Matthew Chapter 22:37-40

Jesus replied: "'Love the Lord your God with all your heart, and with all your soul and with all your mind. 'This is the first and greatest commandment. And the second is like it:

'Love your neighbor as yourself.' All the Law and the Prophets hang on these two commandments."

Galations: Chapter 2:20,21 This is dedicated to my dear husband Dave Stone. He loves this passage and I wanted to place it here for him.

I have been crucified with Christ and I no longer live, but Christ lives in me. The life I live in the body, I live by faith in the Son of God, who loved me and gave himself for me. I do not set aside the grace of God, for if righteousness could be gained through the law, Christ died for nothing!

John: Chapter 14:6-7

I am the way and the truth and the life. No one comes to the Father except through me. If you really knew me, you would know my Father as well. From now on, you do know him and have seen him.

Romans 12:19-21

Do not take revenge, my friends, but leave room for God's wrath, for it is the written: "It is mine to avenge; I will repay," says the Lord. On the contrary: "If your enemy is hungry, feed him; if he is thirsty, give him something to drink. In doing this, you will heap burning coals on his head." Do not overcome by evil, but overcome evil with good.

1 John Chapter 3:1-3 This is another favorite of mine. He still loves me when I am undeserving of his love and one day we will be like Him.

How great is the love the Father has lavished on us, that we should be called children of God! And that is what we are! The reason the world does not know us is that it did not know him. Dear friends, now we are children of God, and what we will be has not yet been made known. But we know that when he appears, we shall be like him, for we shall see him as he is. Everyone who has this hope in him purifies himself just as he is pure.

These verses have been taken from the Women's Devotional Bible, New International Version, published 1990 by The Zondervan Corporation

They have helped me through a very difficult time in my life. I have started attending bible study with Dave and have grown spiritually. I enjoy helping people, being there for them, and witnessing to them. Being there for someone is awesome, we know it comes from our Lord!

Terri Stone